FAST TRAIN APPROACHING...

Breaking Away From Breaking Down

BY STEVE WALTER

'One Million people commit suicide every year'
The World Health Organization

Published by:
Chipmunkapublishing
PO Box 6872
Brentwood
Essex
CM13 1ZT
United Kingdom

www.chipmunkapublishing.com

Proof-read by Flora Wong

Cover Picture
One Tree Hill, Crooklands, Cumbria

Quick and Quiet

There are times when we have to be quiet, to avoid complaint from the children. So I pivot my weight on my elbows to prevent the bedstead from banging the wall and suppress my breathing, avoiding groans only uttering sighs...

Health warning: Some readers may find parts of this book shocking and disturbing.

My thoughts...
By a strange serendipity, I first met Steve standing next to Nelson Mandela's speech on overcoming fear. We were both attending the launch of the *mind out for mental health* programme to challenge stigma in the workplace and the words were engraved in huge letters on the wall. Steve quotes this wonderful passage in his book and they have also played a powerful part in my own life. They provided an immediate ice-breaker to move to a deeper conversation.

I knew immediately that Steve is a man who lives life vividly, creatively, courageously. Someone who uses every experience – inspiring, painful, loving and terrifying – to deepen his understanding and illuminate his spiritual journey.

Here in this book you will find that same searing honesty, creative exploration and bravery. Using poems, dramatic narrative, and diary and medical records, Steve takes us on a powerful journey into mental illness and out again.

This is a deeply moving book for those who have experienced mental illness and for anyone on a spiritual journey. It paints an extraordinarily vivid picture of how it feels to experience mania. And, importantly, it shows how Steve has used that experience to educate people about mental health in the workplace and to campaign for environmental and humanitarian values. It is a revelation and a wake up call – read and be inspired!

Liz Aram, communications consultant and trustee for Mind, October 2006.

My personal view of Fast Train Approaching…

To me, it spoke of the turmoil and confusion that can happen in the human mind with very little warning. It spoke of the comfort to be had from a medium of expression – in this case from poetry. The poetry expresses anger, hurt, frustration but also hope and intense feelings for the human state, and love of the natural world.

The honesty with which Steve has documented his illness – the good, the bad, the ugly and the plain embarrassing is both painful and heart-warming. I know how difficult it was for Steve to acknowledge and eventually accept his illness, for with his artistic temperament he loves and values perfection. The fact that he had what he felt to be a 'flaw' really distressed him, and it was a long, hard journey to travel before he could even begin to entertain the idea that he had an illness that might at any time return. And the thought of medication that might have to be taken for ever just compounded the idea that he was abnormal and unable to manage his life.

The accounts of his memories, his fantasies, his fears (that were terrifying at times), are written in a way that helps the reader to travel the journey with Steve from small boy to sensitive, intelligent grown man. His ability to use words to bring even the most ordinary of things to our attention is, indeed, a gift that helps us to enter into his own particular experience as well as his vision.

I hope that Fast Train Approaching… will be a tool that can be used to help erode the stigma that continues to surround mental illness – although this is becoming less – for such illness is no respecter of persons! It can happen to any one of us at any time.

Jenny Bloomer, Psychotherapist, November 2006.

ACKNOWLEDGEMENTS

I thank my loving lover, Liz, and my family, Mum Hazel, Dad Ted, Brother Tim, my son David, my daughter Amy, my wife Joyce, for everything you have brought to the party. I thank my aunt Jenny, and Chris and Bob the king of the Lakes, my cousins and all who I have loved, friends and family and still love.

To all who offered comments on the draft and helped to keep me on the right lines - I am ever grateful: Liz, Ted and Hazel, Tim, Kyla, Jenny, Steve, Caroline and Padraic.

Also for all my friends at work and in Tunbridge Wells. Everyone else who has also ever offered support, especially Paul and Jenny and those at Ticehurst House. And thank you for reading; I hope you find something of interest here, maybe even of comfort.

I'm also happy to acknowledge the publications where one or two of the poems have appeared, namely The Crack (Links, April 1999), Corpus Christi (the Coventry Millennium collection), In Place of Silence (Poetry South East 2000, BBC Kent website), Skomer (Sycamore Grove Poetry Prize, 1999, Highly commended).

PROLOGUE

I went to the woods because I wished to live deliberately, to front only the essential facts of life, and see if I could not learn what it had to teach, and not, when I came to die, discover that I had not lived.
Walden, Henry David Thoreau, Dover Publications.

Breakdown. Nervous breakdown. Fragments. And in those fragments... something of the truth. I didn't see it coming until the third time around...bearing down on me. I'm more aware now, I watch for tell-tale signs, try to feel the ground ahead of me to predict and prevent that first slip into madness. As if it could happen at any moment.

Sometimes, even an increased fascination with what makes life real, in time and space, is enough to make me wonder – is it beginning again? I think of the cosmos, of galaxies dancing, spiralling across light years. Know the beauty of the last leaf falling, the vixen screaming at midnight, the first snowflake of winter, the eruption of snowdrops. The sun rising. The turning tide. Tiny moments. Momentous ones. The ordinary becoming extraordinary.

Moments when I am intensely aware of the value of things. Not material possessions, but living things. Our environment - everything that has come together to give us life. Aware of our home in the universe, the root of our being... *Mother Earth. Father Sky. Uniting.*
Zuni Indian creation myth from American Indians, The First Nations, by Larry J Zimmerman.

And through it all, an experience of serendipity becoming powerful synchronicity. Living, from casual

13

chance to meaning. From this meaning a new perspective on what it is to be alive. Standing outside the moment. As if you have one foot on the moon...but further away.

Too often we do not give ourselves the time to know what it is just to be...

I am an infant, in spirit. I wonder, will I ever learn enough...? When I give presentations to audiences on mental health and my experiences, I often use this quote, which you may recognise.

So. So you think you can tell, heaven from hell, blue skies from pain, can you tell a green field from a cold steel rail? A smile from a veil? Do you think you can tell...?
'Wish You Were Here', Roger Waters, 1975. Pink Floyd.

I use this to illustrate that our perception of the world, our understanding and the integration of our experience of life is naturally, immensely complex, almost unfathomable; it involves our whole personality, our whole being, our dreams, our aspirations, and yes, our hopes and fears...

OPENING…

Good poetry seems so simple and natural a thing that when we meet it we wonder that all men are not always poets. (November 30th 1842).

The poet is a man who lives at last by watching his moods. An old poet comes at last to watch his moods as narrowly as a cat does a mouse. (August 28th 1851).

The Heart of Thoreau's Journals edited by Odell Shepard, Dover Publications.

I am a poet. I watch my moods. Not only to be aware of the extremes but to register the subtle changes that, may accompany that first slip towards oblivion. I have been close to the edge. I have fallen over …

This account of descent into madness mirrors the clustering of memories: the connections between clutches of neurons that make associations. The flood of neural transmitters across synapses, which at first may seem random. Memory. Association. Out of the random, out of chaos, we draw meaning.

Time. Place. I grew up in Chelsfield, Orpington, which I think John Betjeman put on the map in one of his poems when he said 'the world must surely end in Bromley South or Orpington.' I was two when I moved to Chelsfield in the winter of 1962 to 1963. It was a huge, dark, cold house. After years of work, on my parents' part, it became a vibrant, happy home.

Why poetry?

Why do I choose poetry to represent some of my feelings? I was first liberated into poetry at school when I realised that it didn't have to rhyme. From then on I worked with it to help to express myself. Creativity is bred deep within my family. My father is a poet. My mother an artist. My brother a scriptwriter and filmmaker. My uncle and aunts and many of my cousins are artists too.

Writing is in my blood. Sometimes it hurts so much it burns - the desire to express, to create something beautiful, powerful, out of the moment. To bring the emotion alive, embodied, made real. 'Still life' - dancing.

What is this to be inspired? To be moved by beauty, art, winning performance, ballet, dance, music, painting, sculpture, the human voice, the human body, ecstasy, heights we aspire to...

IN A NUTSHELL
The unfolding of a tale...

I could... rest my ear against the steel...

So what happened? First, let me tell you the story in a nutshell. I'll sketch out the framework, then recreate the complete picture. In 1997, at the age of 37, I had my first breakdown. Two years later, my second. Up until then life had been relatively uneventful, more or less ordinary. It had followed a familiar pattern: school, university, further qualifications, grandparents died. Grandparents I'd loved. I kept fairly fit, healthy, hobbies, cycling, drama, writing, got married had children. My life was normal. At least as normal as life ever is.

The first time, it built up slowly. As well as relationship issues at home, there were factors at work such as the constant pressure to meet deadlines - lunch was the all too familiar hurried sandwich at the desk. On one occasion, I took what most would regard as a 'minor conflict' with a senior manager at work (over a stress research project no less!) as a major, personal insult and this blew the lid off everything for me.

Life began to race wildly. I was on a high. My behaviour was changing. Gradually, more people realised that there was something wrong. At first, as far as I was concerned, I was having one of the best times of my life - I had so much creative energy. Ideas would come flooding in and I wanted to do everything, all at once.

'If anyone is in Christ he is a new creation' 2 Corinthians 5 v 17 - the platform bible poster says...

I was experiencing mania and later delusions as the ideas became further removed from reality, and towards the end, within a matter of weeks, profoundly disturbing. During the last few days I really wasn't making sense. I met with my manager and his boss in a hotel near work. Based on the erratic and unusual behaviour over preceding weeks, they diplomatically recommended that I rest and see a doctor. By this time they'd realised something was seriously wrong. Confused, at the doctors, I was recommended for psychiatric care and, on being admitted I broke down completely: I had experienced 'an acute psychotic episode'.

There were various further diagnoses: bipolar affective disorder (manic depression) stress-related illness, schizo-affective disorder, to name but a few. The symptoms were mixed, unclear. I began to recover in hospital during my first week, with medication. Medication! 'One Flew Over the Cuckoo's Nest' had put me off 'medication' for life!! I was in hospital for a month, and off work for three months altogether. During that time even the first, brief visit by a very caring personnel officer, on neutral ground (a coffee shop near home – I couldn't face the prospect of travelling into London) had me in tears.

Scrambled egg, the pain of breaking shells. Humpty Dumpty dead.

Fortunately my employer took the time and trouble to phase me back into work slowly. After meeting with the personnel manager alone, I met with both her and my line manager, again on neutral territory for coffee in another hotel. With my consent, as well as obtaining general occupational health advice, my personnel manager would discuss my welfare with my consultant psychiatrist. At every stage the options were discussed and agreed with me. We spoke about the job, likes, dislikes, strengths and weaknesses, but there was no pressure to change.

At the first, brief planning meeting while I was off work, in spite of the informal conversation in restful surroundings, I was still very tense and anxious. Although I was lucid intellectually, emotionally I felt very sensitive, vulnerable. After three months sick I was back at work, for only a few hours, a few days at a time to begin with. First I called in just for a cup of tea. To re-orientate. To discover that they were managing without me. That no one was going to take the piss out of me.

I carried on taking tablets for a year (Olanzapine, 10mg). The second breakdown, in May 1999, took everyone by surprise. It happened very quickly, beginning from the moment I woke up, away from home, on a day I was to be lecturing a small class on a course. Increasingly things seemed different, strange. I became afraid, out of all proportion to the usual pre-presentation nerves. I entered another frightening and deluded world. Two days later I was back in the same hospital. A few more days, more tablets and I was sane again. I was keen to return to work, to get back to normality as soon as possible. This time I was only out of work for a month.

Since then I have had more minor episodes. I have worked through them, with the help of tablets: Lithium 1200mg (requires regular blood tests, checks to make sure the therapeutic level is maintained and not exceeded, and checks for renal, liver and thyroid function). Olanzapine 7.5mg (harder to wake in the mornings, more difficult to articulate, combined with weight gain).

when you lie on your back
and cry
tears collect
in your ears...

Listen to the music...among the tensions of iron...the taut melody of steel

What makes us who and what we are?
How old and frail she seemed through the window, sitting in silence, her arms folded against the slightest chill, two bars of the electric fire burning...

What is the nature of spirit? Is it outside as well as within? Is it rooted in something other than time and space? And creativity, are its origins in spirit? I would reflect on these questions on the shores of the turning of the Millennium. They became central to thinking about my personal brand: Making Connections Matter. I was trying to find something that would symbolise my concern for the planet, for spirit and for creativity (see www.makingconnectionsmatter.org[1]).

Throughout our lives, even before birth, we grow in experience through our senses. We are affected by all that we experience - our brains form a million new connections every second of our lives. Our everyday experiences are hugely important in making our brains what they are, and us what we are.

---

[1] *see appendix*

22

Colin Blakemore neuroscientist at the University of Oxford and Chief Executive of the UK Medical Research Council. New Scientist 26th November 2005.

Neurologist Alice Flaherty, assistant professor of neurology, Harvard Medical School, has described her sudden compulsion to write which came ten days after she had given birth prematurely to twin boys.

'In my transformed state I saw meaning everywhere, which made the world radiant, but terrifying. Metaphors came alive.
The Midnight Disease, Alice W. Flaherty.

But always there are distractions. The all too real, delightful and powerful distractions of lust, of sex.

It was too easy, a short skirt, stockings and I was all over her. First the illicit touch: my hand on her thigh, feeling the lace at the top of her stockings. Her black stockings. Suspenders. Her short skirt. My fingers reaching for that sweet horizon: the transition of nylon to skin, of smooth skin to a cropped forest of hair, to the smooth consistency of cream.

Adultery. The name worse than it seems at first. The desire. The lust. The touch.
When it happens, there's no turning back. The contact is a fact that has to be hidden. Kept secret. Each time the secret grows ever more real, builds a tension. Becomes betrayal, weighs heavy, heavier. Until it begs to burst, has to be expelled, excreted, to be vomited up like a poison. And then it is over. Subsides. Leaving behind a deep hollow of regret.

And what of love? It took me far too long to get over first love. For many years, including the years that led up to my first breakdown, I'd wanted to recover something of the love I'd known at the end of my time as a university student. A relationship which ended on New Year's Eve 1982, after eighteen months, when she told me that our personalities were not compatible and I thumped the arm of the chair she was sitting in three times, shouting loud and louder: Crap! Crap!! Crap!!!

All I need

If I were to be honest all I need is what I am.
So why do I long for her, her taste, her touch

Her sex? Surely knowing that I could…
Ought to now to be enough. But I do not want

Only to remember her warmth, her kiss,
Her skin, her smile, her playful laughter.

What I want is to relive those first few weeks,
Months, hours, days, when there was nothing

In the world that mattered more
Than to be together. When our embrace

Broke the hearts of lovers not yet born
And we took what we each had to give

As if it were a child, to grow with us.
All I need is what I am. I am that child in her.

She is in me. I cannot forget. I even remember
The shapes of the bedclothes each morning

As if our every movement were captured
In their soft folds, mounds and crevices.

And I remember the voice of the singer
Who sang to the bonding of our muscles

And limbs, matching the rhythm, and sang again
The day we parted, releasing each other for good.

***

After she'd gone I played *Dire Straits, Telegraph Road* at full volume in my bedroom. My father and my uncle, who were downstairs didn't complain. They understood. The same uncle who, four years later, walked out on 25 years of marriage at their party, the night of their silver wedding anniversary.

But now, for me, another. Her love so complete. Loving her even more deeply...

Number 6. North Street. A One Way sign, pointing skyward, lit up within feet of their front room window. A sign which he almost swings around with one arm as he climbs the final steps to his front door. To her. Home.

There are times when it is best simply to sit, to sit in the sun with a chilled beer, especially in a foreign country. The cold glass between your fingers. Condensation. The first sip releasing you. The alcohol holding you: San Miguel, Kronenbourg 1664, Michelob Lite. Amstel. Peroni. Simple bliss to let it slip in, to overcome your senses.

It is spring, 1997. I have never heard the names of drugs such as Risperidone, chlorpromazine, Procyclidine, and am only vaguely aware of diazepam, but I would come to know, to love and to hate Olanzapine. I write, but not for sympathy. This is nothing clever. It simply happened. An illness. An illness that changed my life. I write for this. To begin to understand.

1997
in which our protagonist discovers…

Alchemy in reverse
What a gulf between impression and expression. That's our ironic fate – to have Shakespearian feelings and (unless by some billion-to-one chance we happen to be Shakespeare) to talk about them like an automobile salesman, a teenager or college professor. We practice alchemy in reverse – touch gold and it turns to lead; touch the pure lyrics of experience, and they turn into the verbal equivalents of tripe and hogwash.
The Genius and the Goddess, Aldous Huxley.

In place of silence

If I were to try to explain how it happened
It would have to do with high tension, high voltage
Breaking the tight line between what is real
And what is imagined. It has to do with boundaries

Between body and soul and spirit. It is about
Aspiration, longing for love, longing to have her
The indefinite beauty who defines a craving heart
The woman within, the muse, playing dice with angels.

And there is always the pain, the slow pain of forgetting
Hidden among the shadows of the haunting past.
Whatever happened belongs to the space between the page
And the written word. It is better unspoken, unheard

Because it fails when it reaches the vibrations of air,
The twisted membranes of the pharynx, the moment

Which is live between the mouth and the microphone
Between the speaker and the eardrum, is best held

Close, except that the silence destroys from within.

***

How to describe it? Breakdown. At first, on a high, completely aware in the moment: imagining I know the true reality of existence in this here, this now, in every moment of my life; feeling my roots make their way among the roots of all life on this planet; sensing the connections which reach back through the atoms of stars, to the beginnings of the universe. It is in this moment that time vanishes and all of the interconnectedness of life merges in the realisation of something greater than the everyday. Something closely connected with every thought, every action, and greater even than death. Here, where we may find our bliss, there is a sense of urgency, of how to value life, not to take it for granted but to celebrate every joy, every heart-felt laughter, in the name of everlasting peace.

We had a railway line at the end of our garden when I was a boy. It is there still. My brother and I and our mates, Andrew and David could climb over the metal fence, by the shimmering tree, the white-beam next door, onto the embankment which fell sharply down to the gravel aggregate of the railway track.

Lying down beside the track I could turn my head to face up the line bound for London, Charing Cross. Rest my ear against the steel. Cold. Listen to the music, the distant orchestra, beginning to play among the tensions of iron, once drawn molten from its furnace. First the strings - violins expand the taut melody of steel. The brass joins in, slowly yet more boldly as the timpani builds the crescendo until the pounding of steel on steel, the crashing of tons of engine and wheels becomes so very real. Do you pull away in time? Or just too late? The rail fuses with your ear - the final blinding silence – crushed in a cascade of rushing metal.

So shifts the breaking mind. First there is a rising tension like that woven into steel as it is pulled into shape, drawn from the furnace, cooling, tempered, cold. Then there is a gathering of electricity, increasing potential difference, reaching a voltage, which breaks through the horizon separating what is real from what is imagined. At the crash the boundaries between body and soul and spirit dissolve, driven by aspiration, desire, a longing not only for love, but for the woman within, the infinite beauty. The Muse. The journey heavenly, random, full of coincidence.

Watch the young boy running to the end of the platform his mother calling his name, the train pulling in…

But there is always the pain of forgetting, the fear of dormant memories that lie in wait, haunting. Sometimes the memory, if resurrected at all, is best left to the written page. Unspoken. Unheard. If you were to bring it gasping, alive to air, to speak it aloud, through the twisted membranes of the pharynx, what truth would it reveal? Remember, reticence, holding it in, traps anger, gradually destroying the heart.

Poems have their magic not only in the silence of the written word, but in the passion of the spoken one.

There are always times when we have to say what we feel. Remaining silent can have a violence all of its own.

Times when it is good to be silent. To listen. To listen to the still small voice. To reflect. To understand. Times when it is even more important to raise the voice from its sleep and to speak out. To place a profound weight to words (as if each were weighed in carats of gold). The glory in being taken slowly, each word savoured before being offered on the white linen of the altar, the open page. Weighed, written then spoken. The human voice connecting through the eardrum of the listener, an audience of souls.

Such a gorgeous picture: she's bending forward slightly over the back of the chair, her short skirt lifting, revealing her stocking tops, suspenders, white knickers…

There were occasional moments in my childhood, before going off to sleep, before I had girls to occupy my mind, when any noises or movements that I made seemed to have been predicted before I chose to make them. As if I had lost freewill. As if my life were governed by some precondition. This was accompanied by a feeling of my centre being shrunk down to the size of a needle, which whirred and spun repeatedly. Something from outside. Whatever I did I could not escape a sense of imprisonment in the tiny moment of time and space, spinning.

Tripe and Hogwash

Later, instead of English, which I loved, I took a degree in Biochemistry and Chemistry because I was interested. Unfortunately, at Sheffield University, I suffered hour upon hour of laboratory work while the art students had the luxury of whole days for whatever they chose to do. Not that I'm bitter! Just a little. Ever since I have been trying to reclaim the inner freedom of the artist. The inner child.

2005

in which reflection is first written…

"It may be that what we call reality is a spontaneous phenomenon emerging like a wave out of some forever unknowable cosmic medium"
Robert Laughlin, Nobel Laureate, Stanford University, New Scientist 9/2/02.

…the brass joins in… as the crashing of tons of engine and wheels becomes so very real…

This story begins and ends on the beach in July, in the village of Petra on the island of Lesbos, in grey volcanic sand. All of time is connected to this moment - like any other - past and future. The roots and connections of the present stretch back to conception and beyond.

A breeze rises with the water. The water curling, arching and falling in tiny explosions of foam, a twisting ribbon stretching the length of the beach.

The sounds of motorbikes, mopeds, scooters, mingle with the hush of the sea and the rattle of the engine of the bus turning into the parking lot off the sea front.

I am in a bar, Café Reef, watching cycling on Eurosport, drinking Amstel lager. My lover on the beach. Lance Armstrong is heading for his seventh victory in the Tour de France. There's a newsflash about a group of women riders out on a training run in Germany. One of the riders, Amy Gillet, is dead. Alexis Rhodes in a critical but stable condition in intensive care. It is reported that the car that crashed into the group of six women racers, was driven by a young woman.

239.5 kilometres Pau to Revel 81.27 kilometres to go. The classements are decided. There's no one in the break away bunch within twenty minutes of Lance Armstrong. Pedals, legs, power, wheels, glide, speed, rock, sway, chain, cogs, revolving, revolving, revolving.

The heat of the sun on rock rises, through the slopes of millions of olive groves, high into the blue-misted mountains. A shimmering breeze sucked up from the sea...

Blood test
"Hello. How are you?" I ask her first. The doctor. We talk about the blood test, the blood I have just had taken. She realises I ought to be tested for sugars because one of the tablets I'm on can contribute to the onset of diabetes. Olanzapine. She pricks my finger mops up the red globule with an indicator stick which slots into a machine. God knows how it works. But I'm normal. 4. Anything up to 11 is fine. Normal. I suggest that since my BUPA coverage is running out that I may need to speak to the Community Psychiatric Nurse. Heaven forbid.

I saw him once before. After I'd come out of hospital in the summer of 1997. He came to my house. Arundel Road. I felt like a once violent criminal, on probation. Him visiting me, in the community. He seemed out of place sitting opposite me, on my sofa, asking me for my history, noting down the sequence of events. His job to keep it on file. Just in case. In case I should need them. They were there to help.

When she says fuck me, fuck me hard, you'd better know she means it…

I visited him at Braeside too. At the fringes of Pembury hospital, Tunbridge Wells. By the woods, where the robins and blackbirds sang. Interviewed, again eight years later, in the place I thought was the psychiatric ward, which was moved to Maidstone. My great grandma had stayed in this hospital. I remember visiting when I was a young boy.

CAMEO MEMORIES

The last of the November sun slips behind the Isle of Wight. Vanishing. Vanishing. Vanishing. Until it is now completely gone. I ask myself if I were to die today what should I remember? What would flash before me? All of this, before it happened...

The house, the dark house, home of trauma aged two. The house I named in my story at school six years later: The Mystery of the Haunted House. Cold. Lonely. I remember being at the bottom of the stairs, the long, dark stairs, before they'd knocked a hole through for a window. It was cold. I was alone. Isolated. I had been moved from a cosy, warm, modern house to this huge miserable, cold space. My parents wrapped me up. Bundled me up warm. Too warm. I threw a fit. My eyes rolling to the back of my head...

...cycling: on two wheels at last, six years old, wild freedom cornering around the side of the house, yet my roaming curtailed, restricted to venturing around the block, and I listened...I didn't break the rules...standing in the school field, twelve or thirteen, writing down the names of lorries passing by on the main road (now a flyover) by Ruxley gravel pits where we used to go bird watching, kids, in the reserve...once we thought we saw a bittern, but probably 'only' a grey heron, the authoritative guide said 'spotting unconfirmed' ...learning birdsong, awake at five a.m. in spring for the RSPB / Young Ornithologists Club at the dawn watch, listening, to note down the first birds to sing, the first song of the blackbird, at least that's what Dad said, not the nightingale or the lark, from then on I learnt to recognise the songs of common birds and grew to love to know the robin, the blackbird, the thrush, the wren, the chaffinch, greenfinch, bullfinch, yellowhammer, corn bunting, nuthatch, green woodpecker, to name but a few, and starling – the impersonator of all of these...

...how every year we went on a summer holiday, early in the morning, getting as far as the first lamp post before stopping so that Dad could get out and go back for something - the windbreak for the beach...cycling over to my Nan's through the country lanes, up Well Hill, past the Rock and Fountain, past the house with the glass observatory, like a small tower overlooking Chelsfield village... conversations over tea and biscuits, tales of the church, of trips to Walsingham, of her childhood, how she brought up two younger brothers while her Dad was away in the army during the first world war, how she would describe London smogs – pea-soupers 'you couldn't see the your hand in front of your face'...granpop, how we rode on the back of his pale blue Ford Anglia along the lanes of Eynsford, with our boy cousins, all jeering as we passed the Witch's House in the hollowed out oak tree, making him drive faster just in case she saw us...climbing granpop's fir trees fighting my way through the forest of tiny, dusty dry twigs my arms scratched, criss-crossed with weals, my face peering out of the tops of the evergreens...

...my Morris Minor, love in the back seat, red leather, the front passenger seat folded down double making extra room for her legs...the policeman who knocked on the window when her foot accidentally caught the light switch at night facing uphill...the white Ford Mexico, three litre, driven to boiling point, coming out of the car park under Kensington Town Hall, the sound of the exhaust reverberating beautifully...

...Amy's Barbie dolls, playing with them, with her only nine years old, as the September sun set over Hurlingham Road near Putney Bridge, how she hated the greasy bacon and eggs in the café on the same morning of her arrival from Florida to London...travelling all around the underground to help find a home for Amy and Joyce...

...reading poems at poetry round in the poetry society at Earl's Court, I chose to read that poem 'how I'd love to fuck the arse of you' not really meaning buggery, just an expression of lust, an amazing screw...sharing a meal with Wendy Cope and friends after the launch of Making Cocoa for Kingsley Amis...walking through Sheffield in my fleece lined lumber jacket, wandering, finding myself in the seedy cinema on the far side of town, seventies porn...

...summer holidays, Devon, Kingsbridge, Dad chasing the batman kite as it headed out across the sands to sea...out with Karen my second cousin for a day trip in Brighton, I always wanted to touch but we resisted...Wales, Ffestiniog, high in the slate mines under a rock hard, blue sky, searing summer heat turning the valleys between mountains of slate into furnaces, silence, no birdsong...Portmerion, the second time around with Alyssia after staying in the caravan – The Art of Finding Things...Loop Cottage, One Tree Hill, meadows, horse mushrooms each covering a slice of toast...balloons one Easter morning, appearing bright and clear over the cottage, breathing flames like the sighs of a contented dragon...the two cylinder Wartburg mixing petrol with oil, driving the lengths of the dry stone walls through the Lake District lanes...

...heavy petting to Knights in White Satin, somehow a conversation about Christianity and my conscience, a naïve sixth-former - we didn't go any further!...with Christine all night , just lying together, moving my thigh between hers, feeling the weight of her breasts, awake as she slept, into the dawn, listening to the chorus, watching the colour of the morning steal over her, how excited I felt, how privileged just to be with her - jubilant...my dear friend Peter who would recite Shakespeare before the English exams: 'Thou art like a man who when he enters the confines of a tavern claps me his sword upon the table and says God give me no need of thee and then by the operation of the second cup draws upon the drawer when indeed there is no need,' ridiculed because of his fair skin, his raging, wiry, blond hair...

...selling glue, driving the A7 to Hawick, flying over the humps in the road, buying Hawick Balls, stopping for a few moments to listen to the silence, a bleat, a chirp, a bleat....Wast Water, the Lake District, resting my feet in the water, eating sandwiches, loving its depth, the huge shadows of the mountains shelving into the lake, almost vertically, taking Alyssia and later Jane over Hard Knott pass...the plastic Samsonite, fractured in the accident - how I was glad to get out alive. How the Skoda pulled out into the outside lane, the fast lane, the overtaking lane, as I was overtaking. How he forced me towards the central reservation. How the car hit it and span. Span round, three-sixty. Sliding along the wet road. Sliding off to the left of the motorway. Crashing into hawthorn trees – one hundred feet the policeman said, suggesting I was speeding-ripping them down as they smashed against the bodywork, shattered every single pane of glass. How the forks of the bicycle I was returning home with shunted into the back of my head, several stitches. How everything stopped and I was facing up hill, up the embankment, my headlights blazing into the sky across the motorway. How I sat bleeding in the front seat of the car I'd passed before it happened, until the police and the ambulance arrived... hilarious that night when her father walked in, my neck brace, her neck brace, her father's neck brace, the three of us together!...

...painting Marie's bungalow inside, woodchip wallpaper, sunshine yellow, a colour she would never really see, Tommy trying to put on tights wanting to get hard enough to pee he said, dicky prostate...Dublin, eating out with him in his suit, sitting with his cousins, roasted by the coal fire in the front room, red legs, backs chilled, the rooms without central heating freezing cold...Dad's stone hot water bottles, filled with boiling water, red hot, incandescent, you barely dared touch them with your toes...

...the cinema with Tara, on our first date, eleven, how I offered her my corned beef and mustard sandwiches, took messages between her and Casey and Sparrow, and there were Hullet and Whitlock who I shared technical drawing with, my page always messed up by marks from my ruler, my sweaty fingers... my notebook grabbed from me by Coombs and Seeley and thrown into the testing pool outside the workshops. How they said they'd found stores of ammunition on a cross country run, how I told my Dad, a policeman and he told the local police and they came to the school and interviewed the boys, it was all made up but they pretended to show the police the place where they said they'd been chased by a man with a gun...dashing from one lesson to the next with Craddock to see who could be first, launching ourselves down whole flights of stairs, skidding briefcases along the corridor to knock other boys down, sliding the same cases off the open decks of red buses so that they raced and tumbled along the ground as the bus pulled into the bus stop... Hawkey saying 'Buttocks' out loud in class, spontaneously each lesson, out of the blue...that moment which I said I'd always remember as a way of marking the passing of time, stepping over the threshold to the canteen...

...my first racing bike, red, with a milometer, the ride into the cold rain at the end of the first week where I was determined to break the hundred mile barrier...Mike Horowitz, Bubble Theatre, Heathcote Williams, his folk-fest poem...The Whale...Frances Horowitz, oracular fields, water over stone, such beauty her perfect choice of words...the Bo-Peep, artex, clouds of asbestos dust, artexing the walls of the gents toilet, painting the bay window, three coats over 90 window frames. Diana. Car washing. Steak and kidney pie. Chocolate gateaux...

Taking our cat Nina from her resting place beneath the bush in sunshine to a family of young children and their cat who'd died of cancer. Nina never that sociable, hiding away, so sad and Amy so upset... watching my heart beat rise to 185 up a hill onto the Hog's Back... going to see York City FC, climbing the York Minster, enjoying Samuel Smiths with my mate Bob from next door... walking to the bus stop for school, through the woods, the same woods that we'd invited Tara to see me naked years earlier, and she would be at the bus stop...

...how I'd run down Warren Road to meet Derek by 7.30 and we'd be the first in school and we'd climb onto the roof of the cloakrooms, using a tree beside them, some 15 feet high to smoke cigarettes, Consulate... on a rowing boat in Loch Lomond at the sales weekend with National Adhesives, convinced that my sales patch was not viable, signing off from the job...Bob Dylan, Sara, at a party in Sheffield, Eccleshall Road, my first time, and everyone else knew the song, sang along, joining in the chorus wherever I could... carrying her, Alice, to another party, Fleetwood Mac Rumours...

...funerals, Gran's, Granpop's, Nan's, them being laid into the socket of the earth...Ken Bird, Green St Green, my bike, Mum's re-sprayed, chippings wrapping up into the Derailleur...taking the engine out of the Morris Minor, selling the number plate 22 TMM...the incident in the chill of the vestry where he'd suggested first aid and wanted me to undress so that he could practice on me, naïve teenager that I was...moments in Bognor lovemaking, black horses...Hildenborough Hall, 1976 The Crusaders a Christian rock group, Nutshell my first album...Tim blowing up a Morris Minor, chock full of LPG cylinders, for the sake of art...

...Poetry Round, Igor Dimont, sharing what we liked about the opposite sex. How she said the rounded, muscular top of the shoulder, how I said my head between her legs. All of us laid out flat as if deep at the bottom of a pool, meditating...Austria, the honey buzzards along the bottom of the flat valleys between the high walls of mountains, surreal with the streetlights climbing up into the sky at night... cousins how once I caught a glimpse of her bare sex as her nightdress blew up as she wafted her sheets up and down playing with her sister...

...Damson and apple jelly, the kitchen in summer as if under siege, moisture dripping down the windows, muslin hanging from the kitchen cupboard, a large round ball of it soaked in red juice dripping, straining through, overnight the colour fading from deep red to pale pink higher up the muslin... chocolate pudding and chocolate sauce, bran pudding, pink pudding like blancmange, rice pink with jam...wasp on my Dad's thumb, how we would watch it eating jam with no desire or need to sting...Windbreak...Appletise before it became popular...

...Mum's big black bike, sturmey archer gears, great for scrambling through the woods, how fast it went in third. Mrs Morris who would slap children around the calves for being naughty for whatever reason... Gill who gave me sponges to play kiss chase - why sponges? An excuse to play... Jane who boiled me in the witch's cauldron with her coven... remembering the girls: Coral, Chris, Melanie, Melinda, Alice, Carol, Diana, Sherry, Katie, Christine, Julie, Jemima, Valerie, Clair, Jill, Jasmine, Mia, Avril, Jane, Elyse...

...finding a round, white stone by a telegraph pole, discovering what it really was as it turned soft in my hand on the summer's day... the girls taken off to see a film together in the last few months at primary school, telling all the boys that it was about Mickey Mouse! They seemed to have been let into a big secret, no equivalent film for us boys.... reading to Marie outside her caravan on hot sunny, summers' days sharing her fascination with Lyall Watson's Supernature and Lifetide...

…the song that pulls all the strings, makes everything so much more alive… the Hot Bread Shop with Paul, all of his motorbike stories, near misses, narrow escapes, thrashing it, the weekend I shared with him and his mates to Silverstone, 140mph past lines of cars which seemed to be standing still - the nearest I had ever felt to death… Kuyokashinkai, him a brown belt, delirious that day he knocked me out while we were sparring, what kind of a kick was that? what kind of a kick was that? I repeated as our tutor drove us to hospital for a check up, not knowing what day it was even though I was looking at my diary…Pink Floyd outside Paris…the Paris bedroom waking to the sound of the traffic rising from the roads around the Gare du Nord standing on the balcony, soaking up the sounds of Parisian life…travelling around Europe on the Inter rail with an AA guide to campsites for directions, camping down in grounds that turned out to be expensive flats, Bruce imagining he had seen sky-lab breaking up… trousers down in the woods to show her, but she wouldn't keep her part of the deal she didn't take down her knickers, the humiliation of her giggling with her friends in the cloakrooms the next day…

…being called bucket, as a nickname, from Walter Bucket… Seaford caravan, huge waves crashing over the shingle, as I lay on the beach happily being thrown around by them, abandoned to the power of the sea. Tim and I throwing a plastic biscuit tin lid to each other as if it were a Frisbee. Practising with my throwing knife which always seemed to hit the target flat. Then my six inch Bowie knife, still a treasure in my sock draw… Hippy Hippy Shake which my Dad had recorded for me on his Grundig reel to reel recorder as one of my birthday party tunes, how I was going to do a wild dance to it, six years old, but lost my nerve, embarrassed, cried, went to bed...

...Seven Mile Beach on Grand Cayman, turquoise blue sea, silver sand, coconuts falling... the grocers, the prohibition notice I served to stop them walking across the twelve foot drop on a plank with no edge protection, no handrail, as they went out the back of the shop to the shed for supplies... the York conference where I played the President of Ecogreenearth, from an eastern European country how I the night before I found the words to set off my character: Shostakovsky Mikailovich Chekov Grad the first words of my address to the audience... spontaneous applause later that day at dinner - for me! ...Nan giving me half pound bars of Galaxy... still trying to wean myself off it... *It's an endless road and I'm at the end of it...*

Northumbria, 16th August 1991: They were out in the field, friends coordinating the texture of earth with three tractors. One cutting the blood brown soil, slicing in, opening it into furrows, turning stubble through the burnt, black surface. Another raking the torn skin, harrowing the turned clay to the delight of seagulls, jackdaws, rooks gathering for the feast of insect refugees and worms. the other rolling out the earth, preparing for seeds... the young lad sitting proud in his insulated cab, cocooned, racing the gears, the four wheel drive Volvo, roaring and bumping over the stubble... red-skinned, tattered vest, his hair swept with the wind, the spray of straw dust and sweat. He is dreaming of Tanzania, when he was supervising his friend's tobacco plantation. Later laughing with his girlfriend, as they spend their evening racing up and *down the track on his motorbike, without helmets, the wind tugging at their hair.*

The decade 1995 - 2005
1995
in which breakdown only happens to others…

Throughout the vital solar cycle the oak-gods are invoked for their aid at the quarterly celebrations of Solstices and Equinoxes. The oak-goddesses are invoked at the cross quarters, namely Imbolc, Beltaine, Lammas and Samhain.

Tree Wisdom, the definitive guidebook to the myth, folklore and healing power of trees, Jacqueline Memory Paterson, Element.

Pumpkin Green
We are celebrating Samhain. Well Halloween. In the name of the druids. An evening of poetry and music in a converted public convenience in Tunbridge Wells - the Forum. An audience of some 70 people. Youth. Poets of the machine chanting their poems to a backing track of rock music. Steve Anthony, a good friend from the early 80s at the Poetry Society plays guitar, sings and reads his own poetry. I am dressed in an ancient wizard's robe, beginning the evening by reciting Dylan Thomas: Death Shall Have No Dominion.

The word druid (Irish drui, Welsh derwydd) is derived from the Sanskrit word veda – to see or to know, or possibly from the word for oak: Gaulish dervo, Irish daur, Welsh, derw. The word for wood and wisdom are very close: Irish fid and fios mean trees and knowledge; Welsh gwydd and gwyddon mean trees and knowledgeable one. The close connection suggests we should think of druid as a 'knower of the woods' or the wood-sage' which would give us a closer feel of what the druid really was – a seer of great knowledge, whose closeness to the natural world put him or her in the position of a walker between the worlds of humankind and the unseen worlds.

The Celtic Tradition, The Element Library, Caitlin Matthews

I knew that after this event, I would move onto something bigger. I'd chosen my goal. Something SMART in management speak: Specific. Measurable. Achievable. Realistic. Time-based. I'd decided to hold an event at the Royal Albert Hall to celebrate the Millennium. A space I'd always admired. Special, big yet intimate, cosy, traditional yet associated with love, with passion: Victoria and Albert. Specific, measurable, time-based but achievable? Realistic? I never questioned it then.

The Millennium. I'd reserved the dates. A week in September 1999. In preparation for the turning of the year. A thousand years. The year 2000. A big deal. A significant threshold. A major opportunity for change. Shifting into a new era. Leaving history behind. Starting afresh. Not just the normal New Year, turning over a new leaf, but a thousand new years, a new chapter, a new book. And it seemed that the transition would be like a digital clock tripping over. The turning of an odometer, gradually realigning from 1999 to 2000. An ending. A new beginning and all the opportunities that offered for reflection - a new start.

Hundred hours

Give one minute's silence.
Listen as the universe turns.

Listen to the quality of fractured air,
To the hollow thud
Of the heart, echoing inside the skull.

Listen to the transient drift of traffic
The catastrophic space between stars
The cavernous tumbling of Earth
As she cartwheels through the heat blast of sun.

Sense the tension between atoms of a grin
Burning, since the moment life began
And is beginning now… and now… and NOW.

Listen for the silence of closing eyes
Which admit the reaper's blade.

And listen, the instant digital time
Flips past ninety-nine
Falls to zero, squares the circle
And we begin again… again… *again*…

***

I was constantly thinking about the Millennium. How could we best celebrate it? How we could celebrate all that is spirit? All that is good that we want to take with us through to the new Millennium. I wrote to Greenpeace, Amnesty International, Friends of the Earth and the Association for Creation Spirituality (as it was then, now called GreenSpirit) who I felt could participate. FoE and ACS came back to me willing to explore more ideas.

23rd August 1995: I believe that the Centre for Creation Spirituality is superbly positioned as a centre of commitment to spiritual values and the future of the earth…Groundswell 99 will be a week of celebration of what is good and great about being alive, being human with a recognition of the darker side of humanity and a resolve to tap new wells of living water for the future…

I met with ACS. The coordinator, Jane, suggested I contact Rob in Bath who was running a company called Groundswell. The same name I had arrived at independently for the event! I visited him in his dark room at the top of his three storey town house, with his tom-tom in one corner and his piling system, his filed papers, piled high in geological timescales. He'd left life in advertising to go freelance and advice green businesses, anyone with an alternative element to their company. He was involved with the local agenda 21, as I was becoming too. (Agenda 21 is an initiative originating from the Earth Summit in Rio in 1992. It places responsibilities on local authorities to undertake consultation with local communities towards minimising environmental impacts).

We got together a small group committed to making Groundswell 2000, as I had renamed it, come alive. At the meetings I would read, or recite, Robert Muller's prayer for the Millennium: My Dream 2000.

My Dream 2000

I dream
that on January 2000
the whole world will stand still
in prayer, awe and gratitude
for our beautiful heavenly earth
and for the miracle of human life.

I dream
that young and old, rich and poor,
black and white,
peoples from North and South
from East and West
from all beliefs and cultures
will join their hands, minds and hearts
in an unprecedented, universal
Bi-millennium Celebration of Life.

I dream
that the year 2000
will be declared World Year of Thanksgiving
by the United Nations

I dream
that during the year 2000
innumerable celebrations and events
will take place all over the globe
to gauge the long road covered by humanity
to study our mistakes
and to plan the feats
still to be accomplished
for the full flowering of the human race

In peace, justice and happiness.

I dream
that the few remaining years
to the Bi-millennium
be devoted by all humans, nations and institutions
to unparalleled thinking, action
inspiration, elevation,
determination and love
to solve our remaining problems
and to achieve
a peaceful, united human family on earth.

I dream
that the third millennium
will be declared
and made
humanity's First Millennium of Peace.

By Robert Muller
Visit www.robertmuller.org

***

I continued with trying to find my own vision. My own personal brand. I wanted something that would combine a sense of time, the Millennium, creativity and spirit. Making Connections Matter was born. This became incredibly important to me. Briefly it means

- the infinite becoming finite, spirit becoming real
- $M^{\circ}M^{*}$ is a huge number, extra-universal
- creative thought, poetry, bringing ideas to life
- mind making sense of the reality we think we know
- bridging the millennium, 1900 (MCM) through the present, to 2100

- connections spanning centuries, grandparents, parents, child.[2]

It is also about linking people concerned for the environmental and humanitarian impact of their purchasing decisions. How these decisions affect other people's lives and the life of the planet. It is about the connections between us which unite us with each other, and with the Earth.

Men's weekends
Many years before I'd noticed a listing for a men's weekend in a circular of alternative events. I was curious, but reluctant. My wife encouraged me to go. Spring '86. Lower Shaw Farm near Swindon. I arrive alone in my three litre Ford Mexico, late on the Friday night. I've had problems with my clutch cable. The AA had to take me home on the Sunday. In between – bliss!

A fantastic sense of community built up so quickly with team exercises which were new to me. Trust. For instance, letting yourself fall backwards with your eyes shut. Trusting that your partner would catch you. Sitting in a circle, sharing the talking stick. Taking it in turns to speak, everyone sharing how they felt, what they valued, how they thought they would grow. Then holding a grapefruit and a banana. At first, hilarious speaking to each in turn, then more serious, revealing deeper emotions.

My tears at some point, early on, helping to ground the group. A brilliant Saturday morning in sunshine.

---

[2] *see appendix*

Silence imposed between us, not a word uttered all morning. Running beside the White Horse at Uffington, running down to Dragon's Hill and dancing to the beat of a drum.

Sunday morning. A ritual. Simulating burial. Covering one of the men lightly with earth, with twigs and leaves. Almost to sleep. As if he had died to the world. Winter. After a while, leaving him in silence, returning to encourage him with song to rise, to break through the earth. The Green Man, born into the spring.

The Green Man featured on another weekend, in Dorset a few years later. 1992. We had been up late around a camp fire. On the Sunday morning we were in a forest glade in sunshine. We were passing round a crown of holly for each to speak. I connected with something deep inside me. Primeval. I screamed. A deep-rooted scream. I cried. Such a powerful release. It felt so good. As if I had found a suppressed inner voice and been reborn through the trees.

One weekend much later, after the turmoil of two breakdowns was over, I was reunited with Alex the group leader, at Hawkwood near Stroud. We were a party of five reflecting on what the Millennium meant for us. What we could take forward. I shared the detail of my earlier meditation in a dried up river bed in Rutland, a powerful personal rite that may have accelerated my breakdown. I cried.

Think of him and his ring tone sounds in the restaurant…

One simple ritual I like on these weekends involves walking out into the surrounding countryside for an hour, reflecting and picking up whatever you find curious, interesting. Fragment of twisted wood, smooth coloured stone, flower. Anything. Then bringing it back to the group and sharing why it is important to you, what it represents. Speaking with it in your hands. This can bring alive many deep associations. Reawaken many dreams. Profound meaning.

'To come to the Teachings in the right spirit you must know and feel many things. You must understand not merely in your mind but in you heart and spirit the impermanence and transience of all phenomena.'

The Buddha was walking with his disciples through a park covered in autumn leaves. He stopped and picked up a leaf and held it out to his disciples and said 'this one leaf represents what I have told you. Look at all the other leaves. They are what I have left unsaid.'

Journey into Ladakh by Andrew Harvey.

1996

Park benches engraved in memory of those who've died…

If only there were evil people somewhere, insidiously committing evil deeds, and it were necessary only to separate them from the rest of us and destroy them. But the line dividing good and evil cuts through the heart of every human being. And who is willing to destroy a piece of his own heart?
The Gulag Archipelago, Solzhenitsyn,

When did things really begin to slide? It may have been in the autumn of 1996, before my environmental exam. 23rd November. How we'd argued in the middle of the night. I'd been snoring, I stormed out of bed at three o clock, sat in a corner on the stairs sobbing, screaming: 'I don't have the answers anymore'.

The black and white photo of her dressed in tight leather holding a riding crop. She is spanking the girl, barely eighteen, wearing school uniform, her mini-skirt flicked up over her buttocks as she bends over.

It could have been later, when I gave a presentation to a group of health and safety specialists on risk in London at the Royal Society of Medicine. The conference: 'A marriage of convenience'. I introduced my slot, the last in the afternoon, with a story about how I had just walked around the park, Cavendish Square Gardens, after lunch before the presentation, as you do, and watched a man with an engine on his back blowing leaves. Autumn. Blowing leaves! Why? It felt like a scene out of Being There. A crazy world. What's wrong with a rake? I asked, rhetorically.

Or was it later that same December when I dressed up as Chief Seattle and read his speech and recited poems.

The earth does not belong to man; man belongs to the earth. This we know. All things are connected like the blood which unites one family. All things are connected.

Whatever befalls the earth befalls the sons of the earth. Man does not weave the web of life, he is merely a strand in it. Whatever he does to the web, he does to himself.

How after Christmas I refused to join my family in Disney World in Paris that cold winter... disliking the commercialism... when I stayed at home and wrote:

A welling up of grief, unexpectedly stirs with me this morning, the baggage of former lives, former lovers, and the hollow silence of Monday morning. A sad remembering, recollection of sunshine, smiles, happiness and endlessly, joyfully, satiated lust.

He thought of words for the beginning of a novel... 'Not everybody likes seafood... Eros is an asteroid... Semen is a kind of glue'... a novel with poems.

It wasn't the search that worried him so much as not finding...the streaks of liquid silver which shot out of him across the desk, the chair, the carpet and even the wall, on postcards from around the world...artistic shots, even a Mapplethorpe now had this protein-aceous liquid hanging from dark skin...'Phwoaarrgh' he'd said, a man of few words, as his body compressed every second of memory and loving into the brief, expulsive ejaculation... there's a novel or two gone... and he set about the place with tissues, making amends, mopping up the sticky tears, which could have fathered thousands, to flush floating, swimming, vanishing down the toilet like any excremental waste... nectar of the gods, such fertility and love mingled, sold down the river, to be digested, meeting their death... no warm womb for those halflings...no silky lining for comfort...no helping hand, no final goal in sight, just a thin watered soup of female hormones gathering in the sewers...

...The beginning of a new millennium is a profound psychological threshold. It causes us to raise our aspirations, our expectations, of how collectively we want to live, what we want to achieve. Many, perhaps the majority, maybe satisfied, at least superficially, by light-hearted celebrations... but others will look for a solid base to build hope for the future in place of despair and uncertainty... it is an opportunity to realise how we might build stronger, healthier lives... how we can rebuild communities, bind together those who share a similar view and have similar wishes for improving the lot of the planet.

Dead sparrow, face up in her garden. Number 13...

1997
in which a fast train approaches…

Can you see what's going on in the trees? The blue and the wind, the blue wind. I've seen that blue wind pass through these same trees only once before…
Nadja, Andre Breton, © 1960 Grove/Atlantic, inc.

But then it might have been that early evening coffee on the 14th January 1997. I was drinking cappuccino with my friend Paul, in Café Sante, 17 Garrick Street, Westminster. At around 7.15 pm as I later noted in my diary. I took another sip of cappuccino which as usual was capped in foam, and I felt something gritty between my teeth. At first, I imagined it was simply an un-dissolved clump of chocolate powder. I reached into my mouth and pulled it out. It took shape in the milky froth between my fingers; it had legs - a cockroach! Dead - thankfully. But a cockroach nonetheless! Horrified. Disgusted. Appalled. Angry. Fuck! That it happened to me. Me - an Environmental Health Officer, who had prosecuted bloody, filthy food premises for less, some God awful kitchens. And the irony, that I should be sitting with my friend, also an EHO.

Wow! Look at the legs on that..!

For some reason, mainly to be rid of it I guess, and against all my training, I handed the cockroach to the employee behind the counter upstairs - giving away the evidence. I asked to see the manager. He had just gone out. I asked for his name. Fred. Fred! Apparently Fred M Zadeh. The Bastard! I rang environmental health the next day and made sure that they went round as soon as possible. I met Fred. Told him how disgusted I was. Wrote to him demanding compensation. He replied, offered my friend and I a free meal! Generous to a fault! Some months later, when I was sane again, I successfully pursued a claim for damages. Fred!

Awake with her all night, through the dawn chorus as she slept…

Not long after the cockroach experience, my first poetry slam. Chats Palace. A Farrago Poetry Slam with John Paul O'Neill. Mock competition. I read Teabag in a Wine Glass.

Teabag in a wineglass

There are many dainty rules
Of etiquette intended to avoid
The incongruous, designed
Not to upset, like picking up

A bone china tea cup between
Thumb and forefinger
With little finger cocked…

Or tipping a soup bowl away
From you, to finish
The last drops with your spoon...

But when the dried lump
Of chocolate powder
Caught between your teeth

Turns out to have legs

Etiquette can go stuff itself
Waiter: there's a fucking cockroach in my cappuccino!

***

A wool jumper, loosely knitted pattern with holes through to her skin the curve to her waist, her soft black skirt...

I haven't tried, but realise it's not the done thing, to cup the buttocks of a gorgeous stranger walking in front of you... I imagine it could be construed as assault, since the girl (or boy) is likely to object. So, get to know them first!

A little black number, short slinky dress, loose broad belt, knee high black boots her legs so smooth, so white…

Contrast: *There's a different world moving and interweaving with this world. Infinite. Significant. It has to do with spirit.*

USA

In March 1997 on a family holiday, after we'd seen grandma in Florida we visited friends in Boston, Massachusetts. Towards the end of the trip, we travelled to Walden Pond in Concord. Water surrounded by woods. April light. No leaves. The trees stirring out of winter. Acres of them. Many young and slender. Encircling the lake. I was captivated. A magical place. Henry David Thoreau. We visited a replica of his hut. His shed. Where he had lived in solitude for two years. His work inspired John Muir founder of the Sierra Club, one of the earliest and most influential environmental movements. I was in awe of the fact that he had spent so many hundreds of days alone there in a tiny hut (1845-1847), simply reflecting on the passing of each day and what it meant for the rest of us.

Just to have taken the time, patiently to describe such experience, to have become so attuned to nature around him, overwhelmed me. What had I done about my concern for the planet? What had I done to counter Man's reckless disregard for the environment? Where was my profound sense of connection to all of nature? I thought that my event in the Royal Albert Hall - Groundswell 2000 as it became known – might make my mark, might make amends. As a young teenager I'd written in my diary about the natural world. I spoke with respect to the tall trees I climbed, so that they might look after me. I still have a book my father bought me called, quite simply, Ecology. It has a marvellous picture of a mountain lion against the sunset on the front cover. For me the picture and the book symbolised all that was precious about planet earth.

On the 21st March 1997, wrapped in the spirit of Walden Pond I wrote: Today, for me, the Groundswell has truly begun. A few weeks later, on Sunday 6th April 1997, even the media announced that there were 999 days to go. I heard it on the radio. The Millennium countdown was for real.

While at Walden I bought Heaven is Under Our Feet, a Book for Walden Woods, edited by Don Henley and Dave Marsh. The cover inspired me. It describes how the Walden Woods Project came to be, to fight off building and development on Walden Woods, a 2,680 acre area surrounding Walden Pond. It consists of essays from some sixty-eight celebrity and other well-known figures, dedicated at the front by Don Henley *'To all those who love and respect the land, the air, the water, and all the creatures who dwell therein'*.

On our return to England, I go to work on my birthday. I had promised myself the day off. With my parents, we go to see Ted Hughes and Seamus Heaney in their reading of The School Bag, in London that evening. A gift from my wife. The combined presence of the two poets moved me to tears. Their poetry reached the root of my being. I wrote to Ted Hughes to thank him, and some months later he kindly replied. A few days after the reading - 19th April is Earth Day. I think of Walden again. What can I do for the planet, for all of life on Earth? What can we all do?

The next day I have a disagreement with my Director General at work, about a stress project no less. I'd prepared for it before I left for the States. I'd worked 'til 8 for several days, which was late for me. He accused the research of being bad science in spite of the fact that it was being organised by a trusted and experienced University. I was furious.

This wasn't a man I could respect. I didn't want to work for him. I'd been there for three years to the day, too long by my account. He ruled the organisation with an iron fist, was never known to be grateful for hard work, and seemed to cultivate an atmosphere of fear. Fortunately I had two engagements that got me out of the office. I had to travel to Edinburgh and then to Sheffield.

Travelling at speed to the twist and flex of steel shackled to the concrete sleepers connected through the blinding rush of the countryside, villages, towns.

I had time on the train to think and to write. I wrote a lot. Almost continuously. Hypergraphia. I couldn't tell at the time, but none of it was making very much sense. I felt inspired. In Edinburgh I was speaking to a group of doctors. One of them took me to one side, had a quick word. She said she'd seen a friend of hers suffer from burnout. She thought I ought to take it steady. In Sheffield I had an amazing experience visiting Forgemasters steel, to see their 10,000 tonne press, forging huge components for cruise ships, prop shafts, propellers. Engineering on a massive scale.

From then on things began to race. I was on a high. It was as if I had made an astounding discovery, that the world was different to what I'd previously known, deeper, richer, more revealing. I was having one of the most fascinating times of my life. Increasingly amazed at ever more incredible coincidences. New life. Happenstance.

And thinking about sustainable development. How to secure the world for future generations, led me to think of waste. Waste from the human. Global. From the refuse ploughed into landfill, or incinerated, to the electricity draining through lights left switched on, the tap left running, to the waste of human creativity in organisations that do not care for the human, the waste of lives, not reaching their full potential, to the global waste of life, people suffering, starving, dying, because of failed politics, wars. And it is the connections between what we do and the consequences that matter. We need to realise the effect we have because

of our decisions, our actions, and their ramifications.
Making Connections Matter.
(www.makingconnectionsmatter.org).

Yet, through whatever circumstances, we may find
ourselves trapped in a certain way of living, a routine
which we feel we cannot escape. And I felt trapped in
my work. Not that it wasn't interesting, but I was unable
to realise where I might go next. What was the next
step in the face of eternal questions - how to save the
world, planet earth? Making connections matter.

Gone away

In your absence
I let my poems
Lie naked on the writing desk
To stare at the ceiling
Without fear
Of rejection

Albert hall
I visit the Albert Hall to walk around the corridors, the
side rooms, to view the stage. I keep my visitor's pass.
Number 70. A memento. I'd calculated that the best
day for the event would be the 22nd September 1999
because that began the hundred days count down to
the new millennium. My favourite date, the 9th
September 1999 (9/9/99), is already booked for the
Proms.

Fat man wading up the hill in the night mist, silhouetted
with his dog, by the orange glare of the streetlight, his
breath in discrete puffs like the smoke from a steam
locomotive climbing, and the dog's piss steaming, oil-

black, running across the pavement, from the lamp post to the gutter.

Church house

Sometimes, on my lunchtime walks from work, I would pass the Church House bookshop in Great Smith Street, just around the corner from Westminster Abbey. I had stopped by out of curiosity once or twice before and not bought anything, but this time I felt elated. I called in. So much potential! I found several books which I was drawn to. I was excited. Everything seemed to have turned to gold. The riches of profound theology. Of prayer in practice. God made real.

Early morning, when huge trucks on a wet road, shifting earth, seem to come crashing out of some terrible future...

I bought Celtic worship through the year by Ray Simpson (£8.99) a selection of different services and prayers centred around creation, the earth, and Celtic saints. I had felt in tune with Celtic Christianity recognising the first saints that stepped foot in Britain.

I bought A New Dictionary of Liturgy and Worship, Edited by J G Davies (£17.50) a substantial tome. Five hundred and forty-four closely typed pages. The liturgy reminded me of processions around our church – St Andrew's - at festivals, feast days. The voice of the priest, the congregation, chanting.

I bought Unemployment and the Future of Work, An Enquiry for the Churches (£8.50) which I felt said something powerful about the social condition for our time. A new politico-spiritual awareness. Inside the front cover I wrote what I felt were important connections: To Stephen from Simon* the Go Between – Father and Son, Corpus Christi 29/5/97. The Big Dream, Creativity, Express, Voice, the Way Ahead for the 21st Century. From the Son who went off to do chemistry 'whatever you want to do but no smoking and hey I don't want you killed on a motorbike.'

*Simon Winter was a pseudonym I'd happened upon which I later discovered to be the same as one my father had used in his writing. Quite independently, I had assigned the name to a spiritual persona, a source of inspiration inside me.

Let all mortal flesh keep silence…
Death shall have no dominion…

Finally I bought a bookmark 'Prayer for the Earth' (99p). To me the church should be actively promoting conservation and environmental awareness as well as the true quality of life…

Prayer for the Earth

O Lord, let the
Earth be a
Growing place,
With flowers,
Grass, and trees,
Where the
Air is clean
And the rivers
Run
Into unpolluted
Seas

O Lord, let the

Earth be a
Living place,
With creatures
Great and small,
A planet filled
With habitats
And for
One and all

O Lord, let the
Earth be a
Loving place,
Where people
Learn to care,
Enough to give
Their children
A world
They're proud
To share

By Jill Wolf.

At the time these poems seemed to me profound, joyful, not like the simple greeting card verse it seems today. I'd spent a grand total of some thirty-six pounds! And I'd never shopped there before. I asked whether they had any other outlets. I decided I could sell their books at St James' Piccadilly. I asked if I could have them on sale or return. They were happy to offer me a discount.

I had hit upon a great business idea! I could make money just buying these books and selling them at a profit in a church only a mile or so away. I could sell them to many churches. I could make a fortune!

> *Synchronicity. When two or three event horizons collide, result in a heightened moment, something other than they were each in their own space.*

In that summer, I visited a management training centre in Rutland. I rose early one morning. I went out for a walk over the nearby country lanes. I was thrilled to simply watch and listen to a skylark rising, singing. In that moment in the quiet of the morning, the creature seemed inspired with the power of an angel. I found a wooded grove within a dried up river-bed. I lay down. I offered myself up to the gods, among the sweet chestnut trees, ash and birch. At that moment I surrendered completely, as if I'd died, giving myself over to another force inside me. Only on rising slowly, did I realise that I was but a few yards from the carcass of a dead badger caught between dried logs in what would have been upstream. It felt as though in some way, I had accepted its spirit. It had entered me.

When I got back to the training centre I felt I'd regressed to a deeper part of my brain, almost Neanderthal. I couldn't operate the coffee machine. I really had to think very hard to work out what I had to do, which buttons to press, much more so than simply a moment's hesitation. As if it were alien to me.

Ruby Sunday
I organised a reception for my Mum and Dad's 40th Wedding anniversary on the 15th June 1997. I booked a couple of guitarists. I'd heard them in a local pub. I liked their music. They sang of people walking in another world. Seymour 60. We had a microphone in a

large ballroom, which I hogged at first. The video clips show me looking gaunt, my words and sentences becoming disconnected. We passed the microphone round for everyone to say something in celebration of my parents' lives together. The tape records a dear friend who was to die only months later.

The date is written in pencil. It is close. Closer. But we can't be sure when it will happen.

Flashback: Tube train

On the crowded underground, Paul nudges me suppressing laughter as he nods to a long gob that someone has coughed and spat, hanging from a swinging handhold above the heads of standing passengers. It grows longer, almost sticks to someone's hair, but misses. It's our stop. We have to leave. Laughing.

She is sketched boldly by his hand. In pencil. Naked. Her legs splayed. Her skin has yet to feel the colour of his brush.

Flashback: Abattoir

…crushed in a cascade of rushing metal…

Dawn. It's clear, from the noises in the lairage that the animals are here. They would have arrived yesterday afternoon. Left to settle. Left to chill. The meat is more tender that way, when they are less stressed. But often, to keep up the pace of production, they run them straight from the lorries, down the ramps, along the concrete corridor following each other, eyes wide. One by one they are let into the metal crate. There is the shadow of a man leaning over. He presses something hard against their head. Cold. Metal. The captive bolt bursts into the brain, splays open, mashing cortex, rendering the beast senseless, then retracts.

Their world turns black and the body drops out of the cage through a metal side flap. Clang. A chain is attached between the tendon and the bone of their hind leg and they are raised on a winch. Suspended from a rail. Once they are off the floor, sometimes kicking, flailing, their throat is stuck. A red rope drops and runs over the smooth, painted concrete floor.

We are here for the inspection. Changing into a white lab coat, a thick plastic apron, heavy Wellington boots with steel toe caps. Round my waist a metal scabbard, sheathing a meat knife and a steel, to sharpen the knife, hanging from the belt. I notice the grease. It's in a thin film over the floor, on everything I touch, the wall, the desk where the inspectors do their paperwork. In spite of grips, of ridges, the boots slide a little on the floor. The grease seems to get thicker as I approach the door that opens into the slaughter hall.

The noises grow louder. The thwack, clunk of the panel the cows fall out of. The whirr of the overhead conveyor as it steadily moves bodies from the pick up point towards the chilling rooms. First the flaying of the beast. The skin cut at the ankles peeled off the back of the body. The severing of the head at the neck. The heads spiked on metal racks. Rows of them ready for inspection. Slitting the body so that the guts spill out. Some for tripe. Or discarded. Then the offal: heart, lungs, liver, running hands and fingers over their slippery skins for abnormalities. The chain saw ripping through the back bone, splitting it in two, spraying tiny fragments of spinal chord.

Sue, another student EHO, said that she wanted to stick them. She wanted the slaughter-man's knife, wanted the power to be the ultimate arbiter of their lives. To stick. To bleed. And I wasn't the only one to feel hungry working there. All of the blood-warm, dead meat. Time for a bacon sandwich!?

Knowing where things have come from. Their origin. The blood and sweat that brought them to you, sometimes across the miles. I want to know whether the meat I eat has come from a happy, free-range animal. One that was looked after, before the last walk, one-way, into the steel and concrete tomb.

Cold hands

Flayed heads hang in rows, spiked on metal racks,
                                                    ready
For inspection. The technique is to hold the tongue,
Long and thick in one hand, and use the knife to
                                                    separate
Flesh between the cheek and the root of muscle.

The tongue twitches as the blade cuts through, slicing
Lymph nodes, tonsils - looking for signs of infection,
                                                    pus.
It's slippery with mucus as it twists in the hand.
Pairs of skinned, black eyes stare, waiting their turn.

On cold mornings, almost comforting to examine warm
Offal, to feel the greasy smooth inner skins for
                                        abnormalities,
The soft sponge of lungs, the ribbed windpipe,
Rubbery liver, the heavy, firm walls of the heart.

Meanwhile, others continue to be hung upside down
                                        and stuck,
Blood splashing from their necks, spilling over
Stainless steel, slipping between drain grates
To gel in chilled vats. Black pudding.

                    ***

In some ways the animals which were still warm, so
recently alive, were less awful, less hideous, than the
cold death of the specimens laid out on the Stainless
steel table for us to inspect at the training centre near
Smithfields, Farringdon.

A is for Abscess

The first atlas of meat and poultry inspection in full
                                        colour, it says
Beside the stamp: Cancelled. Ex-stock.
For the purposes of revision: remember how they look
                                        and feel.

Abscesses in pig spinal cord and pelvis
Often result from bitten tails.

Back bleeding: 'over-sticking'. Note the blood
In the thoracic cavity

And behind the sternum and ribs.

Blood splashing: the haemorrhages occur during
                                        slaughter.
They are most common when electrical stunning is
                                        used,
Particularly when there is a delay in 'sticking.'

Bovine lymph nodes: in some of the nodules
There are specks of pus. This is bright
Yellow in appearance and granular.

Cysts. Sheep brain: this is the cystic stage of the dog
                                        tapeworm
Which causes the disease 'gid' or 'sturdy'. The cyst
                                        has been opened
To show the scolices.

Fluke. Sheep liver: the causal organism of liver rot is
                                        liver fluke.
The typically enlarged bile ducts contain many worms.

Foreign body: pig spleen. Sharp penetrating objects
Such as needles, pins and bristles of brooms
Are fairly common in the abdominal cavity of swill-fed
pigs.

Golden slippers: bovine foetal feet. Note the yellow
Colour and also that the soles are convex.

Infective sinusitis: turkey. The swelling has been
                                        opened
To show the contained pus.

Mandibular disease: 'shovel beak'. Fowl. Note the
                                        distortion

And necrosis of the lower mandibular
Said to be due to excessive dry feeding.

Putrefaction and ascites: fowl. The putrefaction
Is seen as the green colour (arrow).

Tissue mite: fowl. The mites are encapsulated
In the nodules just under the skin.

Xanthomatosis: fowl. The skin is thickened and yellow.
The cause is unknown.

***

Flashback: 24 Waterhouse gardens
It was a routine visit. A council flat. Ground floor
maisonette. The woman that came to the door was
large, very large, and her clothes were wet. She said it
was the leak. That it was about time somebody came
round. Outside it was brilliant sunshine. I followed her
down a bare, dark hallway to the kitchen. She stood in
the middle of the floor and turned, gestured at the
ceiling. But I was looking at the floor. It was grey,
uneven. She seemed to sink into it, as if it were a bog.
I gradually realised in the gloom (the light had blown
because of the leak she said) that the floor was
covered with layer upon layer of newspaper which had
formed a kind of deep, papier mache mulch, soaked as
it was, completely soaked through.

All around the room there were pots, bowls, jugs. They
were set to catch the water. Water that was dripping
from the ceiling and had evidently been dripping for
weeks. It was an abstract, discordant music: the drips,

their scale of harmonics ringing out in the assorted kitchenware.

She had difficulty explaining what had happened, forming sentences. She let the room explain. She took me into the dining room where her husband was lying in a bed in the corner, shaking. He could hardly speak, couldn't get up. Evidently, he had Parkinson's.

They had abandoned their bedroom. I looked into it, from the door to one side of the kitchen. The bed had sunk through the floor, each of the legs puncturing rotten floorboards. On one wall, high at the join with the ceiling there was the thick taproot of a young tree growing into the room. Judging by its size, it must have been growing for years. I later discovered that the dripping water was from the storage tank overflowing in the empty flat above. It wasn't the first time she'd tried to raise this with the council. Nothing had been done.

Flashback: Poetry circle
We are near the end of a weekend of reading and writing at Canterbury University. Poetry. We are reading in the round, sharing our writing, reciting poems in turn round the circle. Such a spread of ages. At 23 I'm one of the younger ones. Next to me, Tom, past retirement, over 70. While someone is reading to the other side of me he coughs, splutters, then throws back his head. Quicker it seems, than we can do anything, or realise that anything is really wrong, there is a long sigh, and a rattle from his throat, as the last of his breath expires. Next to me. I don't know what to do. Someone calls an ambulance. Someone loosens his collar, with help lays him on the floor, as if to recover. Paramedics confirm what we have not dared to utter.

Flashback: Bag Lady

It is a clear, bright sunny spring day. An official looking bunch of people is gathering outside a house in a street in Clapham. 32 Eden Park Road. The home of the bag lady. She has been reported pushing a horizontal hooded pram collecting whatever she finds of interest on the streets. Rubbish. We have had complaints of mice from the tenant sharing the house. We have a warrant - I got it - my first experience of court, as a newly qualified Environmental Health Officer. Wandsworth Magistrates' Court. I am proud of it - my warrant under the Prevention of Damage by Pests Act 1949. We could force entry if we need to. We knock first. We wait, seven of us: a locksmith, policeman, social worker, two environmental health officers, two pest control officers. This time, after some persuasion, shouting up to her as she leans from a first floor window, she lets us in. The hall way is cramped. There are bags scattered around, full carrier bags of all shapes and sizes. The door into the front room when pushed hard opens onto piles of jumble, old clothes, old boxes, containers, newspapers, plastic bags, every variety of rubbish, even remains of food, piled easily five feet high. Through it all the rank smell steals over the senses, so strong that taking a breath, I felt I might drown. Everywhere shopping bags of rubbish. The dining room floor is rotten. The kitchen cooker is black. Burnt pans. Rubbish. More rubbish.

We find our way upstairs, stepping over all kinds of sacks, into the front bedroom. There is a narrow pathway between towers of plastic bags full of indescribably useless bits of discarded modern life. At the end of this artificial corridor we find a narrow single bed. In the bed a boy, timid, maybe fourteen, half dressed, with a shock of black hair, who looks at us blankly. Has he ever been to school? Has he ever gone outside? How has he grown up in this? The inside of a refuse truck, a dustbin lorry! It's our job to clear the house. We begin. The policeman and locksmith have gone. The social worker has some serious thinking to do.

The journey begins
Monday 21st April 1997.
The guard announces that our train, which would normally have gone through to Charing Cross, is to be terminated at London Bridge because of a security alert. The IRA has set off coded warnings at all the country's main railway terminals.

I get off the train at London Bridge, and, because it is such a beautiful morning decide to walk to work along the embankment. It's a good couple of miles. I will be late but what the hell, there are more serious things going on.

The electric sounds of the grackles like shiny blackbirds, silvered black metallic magpies, calling from the trees, saw-grass, heat, alligators dreaming in the lakes, beneath the radiant sky…

He crosses the busy Borough High Street to Southwark cathedral which is being cleaned, surrounded by scaffolding. A loose, white, plastic sheet flaps in the breeze. A few weeks later, he would do this walk again. There would be a beggar sitting at the entrance to the cathedral grounds. He would hesitate, walk by. After a few paces, he would stop, turn back, hand something to the beggar, with an apology. A ten pound note.

I have only a penny
If I were to give it to you
It would be an insult

      stop, think again

I walk away then turn
And hand him a tenner
To ease the pain.
               (Friday 30th May 1997)

Today he continued to walk between the narrow alleyways, passing the Golden Hinde and the Westminster Palace, Bishops' Palace, Clink Street and pausing at The Clink. He struck up conversation with the lady at the turnstile. The place was being run by Rankin, the surname of his dead step father.

He passed the Tate Modern nearing completion and the fenced space on the embankment, set aside for building the Millennium Bridge.

Eventually after following the Queen's Walk along the South embankment he crosses Westminster Bridge - a route he once always took to work from Waterloo. He passes Westminster Abbey, promising himself to revisit the place and have a proper look around, rather than simply kneel in prayer.

When he took the walk again in May everything suddenly seemed clear to him. He thought this would make a fantastic trip through time, admiring the architecture - a walk for the Millennium. Years later he would discover, in the year two thousand, that they did create a Millennium walk through these exact same streets.

Loop cottage

Set in the lowlands bordering the south-eastern tip of the Lake District, a stone's throw away from the M6, yet silent. Loop Cottage, Crooklands. Close to one tree hill. You could see the tree clearly from the motorway in the middle distance when passing Farleton knot, the first great hill next to this stretch of road. A rocky limestone outcrop. Loop Cottage. My second home. Part converted from farm buildings, an old barn. Cosy and loving. My brother and I stayed when we were young teenagers. We met our cousins for the first time and fell in love. The two eldest girls Jo and Becca, closest to our age, then dear Lucy and George.

A cooking range with an open fire that was nearly always burning. Logs and coal. In the early days a weaving shed sheltering a loom with a shuttle weaving, crashing, warp and weft. Later, it became home to my uncle's graphic arts studio. Fern Art. Shelter for bikes, a ping pong table. My uncle left my aunt on the night of their 25th wedding anniversary – the night of their party. Afterwards, the weaving shed stored furniture for years. Then my aunt had a vision which I shared, it would become a meeting place for dreams. It was insulated, revived, opened for peace dancing. Dancing circles, singing in foreign tongues, accompanied by a guitar. Sharing food afterwards. An oasis of peace.

One tree hill

We play beside dry stone walls
run the paths
beaten through grassy fields
and skip, on switch-back lanes.

In this huge country, the vast acres
of gorse, heather, limestone crags
and mountains threaded with necklaces of stone
are backdrop to brightly coloured dresses, dancing

circles, and you, mother to our cousins
laughing with the girls' laughter
spinning your own unique sunshine
giving yourself, to make Loop Cottage home.

And we grew with the flame
of their changing, our sleep barely
disturbed by the flight of curlews, their song
like hands, rippling the skirts of dawn.

In these hills, I crossed freezing water
with my Uncle. We shared whitened feet
pulling on our warm, thick socks
together, like men do
before I learnt the word divorce.

***

We visited in the late spring of 1997. I was high. Highly
charged. Emotional. So glad to be there. Tom, a friend
of my Aunt's helped to design the logo for *making
connections matter* with me. It was simple. Beautiful. It
contained all I wanted to say about time, the
Millennium, creativity and spirit. (See the appendix for
the story of what M^{c}M and *making connections matter*
mean.)

On our return south from Loop Cottage to the outskirts
of Bradford, I had been noticing the number plates of
cars on the motorway. I'd decided that those with the

prefix 'M' were owned by MI6. It didn't occur to me that this was simply the latest registration, and wouldn't it otherwise be just a tad obvious!? I flashed an M reg car that had been playing tag with us, as we were travelling at the same speed. He flashed back as he left on a slip road, confirming my theory.

In Bradford, for some reason I was boiling over, screaming at my wife as we walked through the high street looking for a place to get a bite to eat. We eventually found a small grassy slope beside a road to have sandwiches. My son had been upset, crying at our row. One of our apples lost its resting place, rolled down the little hill into the road, much to his delight, our laughter. We rolled another apple, tomatoes, breaking the tension…

In a service station sitting down for tea, I noticed that a man sitting with his back to us had a mark like a scar on the back of his head. I confided in him. 'So they got you too – a chip inside your head, that's how they know everything about you.' He turned and smiled. My family disowned me in embarrassment. I carried on talking to the man, he humoured me…

Westminster Abbey
One of his favourite places is St Faith's chapel, deep in the heart of the abbey. It can be reached by a large, heavy oak door direct from Poets' corner beside a sign which says 'for prayer only', or through a smaller door by the Chapter House. He used to avoid the main entrance and the tourists and enter the abbey from Dean's Yard through the cloisters in the old monastic quarter, by the Chapter House. Now there is always a warden on duty, who you have to ask for permission to step inside the south transept from the cloisters. Few

people ask to visit the chapel for a moment of private prayer. Few people enter without paying the tourist fare.

St Faith's is a special place for him. It's part of the abbey which was rebuilt in the 13th Century, by Henry III. He loves to be alone there, to kneel in the silence. The huge height of the stone walled room above him. A perfect place for prayer. Occasionally a tourist who does not read or understand the sign opens the door just to see inside. With the door open, he hears the hollow echoes of muted voices and footsteps in the whole of the abbey, and the whispered mutterings of those nearby. He resents the intrusion. Returning to silence he adores the strength and resoluteness of the stone, this space in the heart of London, which has stood for so many hundreds of years. Vast. Spiritual. Filled with the spirits of the dead. You could feel them on cold days drifting through the cloisters. Walking over the Black Death stone. Benedictine monks.

Church had seeped into his childhood. St Andrews. Confirmed. As a young boy he donned a black, ankle-length cassock, a pleated white, waist length cotta. He'd been confirmed as a teenager. He and a friend had shared leather armchairs at the vicarage where the vicar talked to them for more than an hour every Sunday after church, for months.

First, he was a crucifer carrying the crucifix, leading. Then acolyte. Bearing a candle. He helped the priest in and out of his chasuble before and after the sermon. Saturday mornings he would cycle down to Orpington, from his home in Chelsfield, to get to the church by ten past seven to prepare for the service to start at 7.30. Usually, it would be just him and the vicar. No one else was fool enough to share communion at that time on a weekend. The vicar did the same everyday. High church. High Anglican.

This lunchtime, he decided to have a proper look around the abbey, as any tourist would. He found a guide, an old lady, who was the spitting image of his maternal grandmother, his Nan. She showed him the stalls of the knights and the Battle of Britain chapel. She led him past the graves of the original kings. He cried at the depth of history. He thought of all the lives of those who'd sweated to construct the building. All those who'd died, either unknown or shrouded in stone for posterity.

St Matthews
Later the same month he visited St Matthew's church in Great Peter's Street. He arrived just as the lunchtime service was about to start. It was Corpus Christi a day of the Christian calendar which was one of his Nan's favourites. He didn't know much about it, save to say that it had to do with God becoming flesh through Jesus Christ. Special. Incarnate. The music from some of the Kings College choir moved him deeply. He began to cry. He had no tissues. He asked the man sitting next to him and he was given a cotton handkerchief which he used to blow his nose, flushing his sinuses of phlegm. He offered to return the handkerchief. Needless to say, he was politely refused. He was still crying as the priest held out the unleavened bread for him to take for communion.

Corpus Christi

He kneels, as if he has witnessed slaughter,
Sobbing, while other communicants stand
Holding out their hands for the Body of Christ.

The white cotton handkerchief he borrowed
Is soaked and stained with silt
Drained from the channels in his skull.

For a moment the power of Christ crucified
Rings true and he is overcome
With the resonance of violent compassion.

His dead grandmother kneels with him.
They walk through Westminster Abbey
Treading on generations of the English monarchy.

The wafer passes from palm to lips,
Entire moments pour
Through her fingers like liquid air.

Likewise, after supper, He took the cup.

***

'It's not time to make a change just relax take it easy'

I hear these words for the first time and I am transported. Another world. 'I know that it's not easy when you've found something going on'. The day takes on a different dimension as if I can see through to the roots of things, their connections interconnections and coincidences... 'all the times that I've cried keeping all the things I knew inside'...

The red-bearded man sings, playing his guitar at the foot of the main escalator, at London Bridge Station. I am carrying a huge overnight bag with me over my shoulder. It feels as if it's getting heavier and heavier. As if it's the burden of a pilgrim growing with my sins, or a cross weighed down by the sins of the world. I think he is homeless, the singer, yet he sings with such passion. His gravel voice licking its way around the tune and the lyrics. He smiles as I ask him who wrote the music. Cat Stevens. Father and Son.

I buy the album, the Very Best of Cat Stevens. I play it over and over, especially that track. I play it for my parents when they arrive one day. I cry on my father's shoulder. This is how it was in childhood. Told to listen. And yet God, how I love him. Father and Son.

Friday 13th June
Work, arrange an appointment for me with an occupational psychologist, Dr Mike Kaplan. I visit him in Longmore Street SW1 at 2pm on Friday 13th June. I mention that I have never worked anywhere for more than three years before, and say that it is about time I moved on. We talk about acting, writing, poetry. We talk about job options, how it would be difficult to re-train, having got so far in my career already, although I would have transferable skills, such as giving presentations.

The following week on June 17th I see Gerard Benson (who was one of the founders of Poems on the Underground) and the Apollo Chamber Orchestra in St Martin's Church:

More beautiful a combination
Of poetry and music
I cannot imagine.

I am in tears in the audience, such a powerful, moving performance. I knew Gerard from a writing course more than ten years earlier at the Poetry Society. He knew that things weren't quite right with me. He understood mental health. He seemed concerned. I'm not sure why, but one of his friends gave me some money, I think to get the tube home because I said I was short.

A few days later, on 20th June, I buy a cassette of This Sceptered Isle. It seems to say something of my experience, conscious of Victoria, her love for Albert, grieving his death. The Albert memorial. The Royal Albert Hall. The Millennium.

So many thoughts
So many dreams
So many visions

Sprinkle them
One by one
Like confetti
Across the page.

Media

I am laughing so much at so many adverts. It seems they realise something of the sense of the moment and how things are changing. They speak to the deeper parts of me, as if they are in on a joke. They play with archetypes, profound symbols, they get to me, make me laugh out loud at the irony, selling with psychological tricks. And the radio. I hear phrases in news reports, documentaries which speak to me directly. I imagine they are real messages to me, specifically to me and my situation, because of the coincidences between their stories and my reality. They are talking to *me*. They want *me* to hear. And I am singing my own composition.

Spinning in my head
Like a dream without a city
Lies a man with the answer
To the turning of the day

22nd June 1997
We have to find a way.
We have to be true
To ourselves… we have
To dream to understand.

Like King Canute
You can't fight a rising tide
Neither can you
Fight a dying sun
You have to greet
The new day
With open arms.

True connection with this world is through the tiny magic of today.

Commuting
Walking to the station I nod and smile and say hello to all who seem to be in on the act. To the decorator half-way down our street. The old man walking his red setter. The station manager. I am writing notes busily,

furiously. Crossing Parliament Square, I stop in front of the statues, Lincoln. Something inspires me. A thought. A quote. The moment. I am late for work again.

On the journey home, rocking from side to side, the other people in the carriage are making indirect references to me in their conversation. Almost anything anyone says holds some significance for me. In one way this is comforting, it's almost as if I am being looked after. But I cannot work out why this should be. Why should everyone be looking out for me? Am I really special? Are they aware of this other world, where everything is so much clearer? It's as if I am in a sketch where everyone knows what will happen next, except for me.

Moments when he became acutely aware of cunt. Cunt, on every gorgeous woman he saw. Cunt on those less gorgeous. Cock hungry cunt on all of the girls and women around him. The sexual power of cunt. Delicious, horny cunt. And how he wanted it. Wanted to share it, to bring it alive at his fingertips, to pulse, clasp and unclasp, to be tight around the thick of him.

Surgery
On the morning of the 25th June 1997, he walked into the doctors because he knew there was something wrong. He had been told to. His bosses had suggested so the day before when they met in the quiet of a hotel club room near to the office (he'd told them about Groundswell 2000). He'd stood with his immediate boss on the bridge over the lake in St James's Park facing Buckingham Palace. He said, 'Don't you just feel you could step onto the water and walk on the

surface?' Mallard. Coot. Tufted Duck. Red-crested pochard. His boss steered him towards the hotel.

But it wasn't just what they said that prompted him to go. He didn't feel right. He felt as if there was a shadow trailing from the back of his head as if something dark were clamped there, with a long tail - feeding. The receptionist told him to go into a room to rest and wait and a nurse would see him. She did, she was concerned because all he could say was that he didn't feel well. He looked at the numbers on the scales beneath his feet. He seemed to be growing lighter by the minute. And then the doctor saw him. It felt like only a few moments but afterwards he learnt that he'd actually stolen nearly an hour of the doctor's time. The doctor arranged for him to see a consultant psychiatrist.

He looked at his wrists, studied the way the dark hairs sprung up around his watchstrap, how they petered out to finer hairs as they ran up the back of his hand. How distinct his veins were that carried their warmth back to his heart.

Ticehurst
His wife took him later that evening to Ticehurst hospital, near the village of Ticehurst in East Sussex, bordering Kent. It stood, huge, white in the low evening sun, with high, ornate parapets. He met a psychiatrist (who was to become a good friend) who asked him apparently straightforward questions. Simon thought he gave straightforward replies, but the look on their faces told a different story. He was invited to stay.

The tick of the Waterhouse wall clock, enhancing the silence of the reception, the magnolia walls, wide mirror over the mantel-piece, sunshine spilling through the windows…

The only spare room they had available was a mother and baby room. They left him there. It was cosy, comfy, pink. He felt safe, protected. He could now be everything he wanted to be. He'd lost all inhibition. He loved standing naked and erect. He masturbated, looking at himself from three different angles in the vanity mirrors on the dressing table. He thought when he crouched down on the floor, that he could clearly see the individual sperm he'd spilt on the carpet when he came, swimming. He was delighted. He told the nurse when she came in, what he'd found.

Gorgeous tits…

They gave him pills. He imagined that he was somehow special that the new faces of all of the nursing staff who popped in to see him, in turn, to check every fifteen to thirty minutes, were enlightened visitors from the future congratulating him on his success in his life, as if he had really achieved something. Something big…something spiritual…

If you had told me thirty years ago that I'd still be wanking at 45 I never would have believed you…

Later that night, he realised that some of the nurses were prostitutes. At first he thought he would experience a little, erotic S&M. He was excited. Then he discovered they were out to hurt him, real bad. He was to be punished. Punished for the sins of the world. Punished for all man's inhumanity to man. Punished because he was responsible for the terror, the suffering and torture throughout all time. He was going to be born backwards through the ages. He would have to suffer with everyone who had ever suffered until the first light of history. He would bear the pain and suffering of the world. He was to be held to account for the anguish and murder suffered by millions of Jews. He was their atonement. He had to experience their agony.

At the same time he was convinced that he'd discovered the question that led to God creating the universe. The Devil tricked God into saying 'No'. God had not wanted his creation to be able to deny him. When he said no to the Devil the world was suddenly awash with the shadow, with denial and deceit. Now there was pain in a once pain–free world, and there would be suffering. God suffered. He screamed. All was not perfect. Yet it had to be so. They came in when he raised the alarm. He pressed the alarm. One of the nurses, a tall, burly man showed him the nib of a biro, convinced him, that this could inflict pain. That it would be a bad idea to keep raising the alarm. It would be painful. He was terrified.

He was convinced that he was going to die in the Royal Albert Hall. That he would be shot there, while staying in room 101 on his birthday in the next Millennium.

He imagined rain. Rain pouring in through the ceiling of his home. Tears of his wife. Rain pouring through the ceiling at his work. Tears of his colleagues. And rain flooding London, Westminster. Tears, connected to the news later that summer, one Sunday morning when he woke to hear that Princess Diana had died. The tears shed throughout the country, condensed in London.

The tears of the mourners who lined the route of the funeral procession through Westminster.

The next day they showed him around the carpeted corridors. He noticed the fire doors. They seemed to be arranged strangely, as if they were somehow there for keeping people in, not for ease of escape, in case of emergency. Some Georgian glazed doors, not exit doors, were controlled by keypad. As if they were there to diffuse tension, for anger to be released, for fire to escape. Fire Exits. To protect those within from those outside.

Nobody could understand how the ordering of the meals worked. Each morning they would complete a sheet saying what each of them wanted for breakfast, lunch and dinner the next day. Of course by the next day you couldn't remember what you had ordered the day before.

'I love the feel, watch how it swells, fills and rises…'

He was introduced to the lounge. A soft, pink-carpeted floor, rose coloured walls high ceiling with a small, courtyard off to one side where people could smoke. There were several deep armchairs and an equally comfortable sofa. In the corner there was a small drinks machine with trays of cups and saucers, clean and dirty, separate. Looking around he found it hard to tell who were the patients, who the carers. They blended in. Nothing was rushed. There seemed to be a steady, relaxed air about the place.

'I love sucking cock. I love giving head. It's kind of like an art form you know.'

All the days are full of glorious sunshine. It's June 28th. At about four or half past in the morning, he is wide awake. He wants to get out into the open air. He walks along the yellow corridor to the staff office where he asks a man who seems to be the only person on duty, to be let out for a while. The duty officer, not a big guy, says no. They stand arguing close to the exit door. About a metre away.

It's an easy thing to do with a little practice, a side-kick. If you stand a couple of feet away to one side from what you want to hit, depending how tall you are, then raise your leg nearest to the object so that your knee is level in front of you then swiftly, hard and powerfully extend your leg rapidly, horizontally, as if straightening completely and kick sideways through the object you are aiming at. Chances are you will inflict some damage.

Needless to say, he did a side-kick to the back door and amazingly enough it opened. He was out. The duty officer went back to his office, presumably to phone for help. Determined the patient took off on a walk around the grounds. He was planning his escape. He happened to find a monkey wrench lying around on a small building site to the back of the hospital. Then he came across a couple of old saloon cars, an old Ford Cortina and an Opel Kadett near to some of the other hospital buildings. To him it looked as if they were both wrecks. He decided that to make the best job, he needed to take the front of one car and join it to the rear of the other. He started prizing open the lock of the Cortina, levering the handle with the wrench.

After a while he realised he needed other tools and thought perhaps he could find someone to help. He walked back along the drive, across the gravel, to the front entrance. It was nearly half past five. The front door was locked. As he was pulling on the door, trying to tug it open, a police car drew up silently. From the front, the faces inside were hidden behind the sky reflected on the windscreen.

He went over to the police car and tapped on the nearside window with the monkey wrench. The police officer in the front seat didn't look at him but kept staring straight ahead. Another police car arrived, silently. He found himself talking with an officer saying that he intended no harm, when together the others jumped him from behind grabbing his arms and legs bringing him to the ground. They pulled down his trousers. He screamed, fearing rape. His buttock was jabbed with a needle and he relaxed. They bundled him back to his room. He couldn't resist. All under a royal blue, morning sky.

...the rail fuses with the ear...

When he came round he discovered that they had written out a formal section under the mental health act to protect him from himself. He had been sectioned! He was given the chance to appeal. But by the time his appeal was to be heard, he was better and the section had already been lifted...

The drugs made me slow and dopey especially in the mornings. But I often took the opportunity to run around the grounds along the footpath, beneath a tunnel of trees. At least, afterwards, I felt that I'd achieved something: puffed out, exhausted for a while, heart beating quickly.

One of the drugs I was prescribed after the breakout, after being sectioned, was Risperidone. But I began to itch. After a couple of days I'd come out in a rash. I was itching all over. It was as if I were covered by tiny bites. I was so grateful to one of the supervisors. He was tall, massive. The same nurse who'd frightened me over the nib of the pen. Friendly. Roger. He had huge hands. His huge hands rubbing calamine lotion into me, the milky solution I used to have smeared onto me as a kid to treat sunburn. Cool, drying pasty white, to soothe the irritation. Such relief.

Windbreak

He'd hammer the wooden rods into the shingle
With a rock the size of his palm and the wind would fill
The striped cotton: green, orange, yellow, brown.

Once punctured, the blue camping Gaz cylinder hissed
Into the burner, the flames tickling the base
Of the aluminium kettle. Mother would open the
                                      Tupperware

Box of sandwiches prepared that morning in the
                                      cottage,
While the sea would rise and fold, easing itself

Between the pebbles, inviting us back in. We would
Have to wait an hour before the food went down
And we could swim again. The whistle brought
                                      scalding tea,

Our skin turning beneath the sun, pasty white to red,
                                      burning
Between the sheets at night, in spite of cool, calamine
                                      lotion.

__The Book of Common Prayer__, everyone should have one to take with them everywhere, to dip into to quote from, to family at breakfast, to friends on the train, to work, to traffic wardens, shopkeepers, to lovers in the park, skate boarders, undercover policemen…Dearly beloved…We do not presume…Amen

I used to love the chance to walk into the village. Ticehurst. Summer. At first I had to be accompanied. But then, when they recognised that I was returning to normal, I could go alone. The leaves singing in the dry heat. The village sign occasionally swinging beside the road. I walk past the coach station, past the tea shop, the oak hut of the bus stop, the grocers, the post office, to the second hand bookshop by the church. An old book on the millennium in the window. Two huge yew trees standing in the grounds, creating an archway. The cool silence inside the church. A brief moment for reflection, prayer.

Ambling around the grounds with my parents, their shadows walking tall in the long evening light…

Then a few days before leaving the hospital I was allowed to travel home on a bus by myself and stay overnight, phasing myself back into what had been normal. An adventure. Real life. Handing over the coins to the driver, asking to go to Tunbridge Wells, by the station. Like being a kid again but this time amazed at the everyday, by what people accepted, getting on with their lives. People in my street accepting me, some saying how they'd felt wobbly several times, had almost ended up inside.

The crack

Even the seasons seem to shift like seismic faults
Winter-spring, spring-summer, and weather
Fronts cascade leaving only a shared skin

Of refraction, air-water, water-glass.
And the moment feels like yawning steel,
Inner surfaces slide friction free, their tension
immiscible.

Personality set to disintegrate. Seconds mark the
borderline, the threshold between sane-insane,
Free-captive. And I think of rain falling on limestone

Watch how it freezes, how it splits the rock
Breaks open the skull of a mountain
Makes me listen to the molten brain within.

**

MEDICAL RECORDS
Date of Arrival 25th June 1997
Date of Departure 23rd July 1997

Presenting complaints
Admitted for investigation and assessment of recent
weight loss, perplexity and polydipsia.

History of presenting complaints
Difficult to get a clear history from patient until late into
the admission. In essence he was able to explain that
in January 1997 he had coffee at a café in London and
almost ate a cockroach. This incident appeared to
upset him greatly. He even wondered at one stage if
he had PTSD from that incident. However, it is clear he

became preoccupied with this and did complain to the manager and did send the Public Health Officer round but he still retains to this day ideas that it wasn't properly dealt with and that he would like it to be dealt with as a matter of principle rather than trying to gain something for himself. Following this, he feels that there were no real problems until after he returned from his holiday in America on 14th April 1997 – he recently had a birthday. He also felt very unsettled after arriving.

There was an incident where he had a meeting with the director general of the company he works for which left him in a lot of turmoil in his internal life. He felt that he wasn't being listened to by the director general, and for the following week and a half he found himself going through a period of intense revaluation of his whole life. He described it as taking stock and that if his life was on a computer he thought that he was putting a lot of it onto a 'hard disk' and that he had got rid of a lot of it and that if he had had a silicon chip he would have downloaded it. Since that time he describes that people have been reacting oddly towards him.

Certainly, his wife reports that he has lost weight and became increasingly perplexed over the next three months, being also increasingly out of touch with reality. He was also drinking excessively (not alcohol) and expressing some bizarre ideas. No suicidal ideation on admission.

Past psychiatric history
At the age of 12 he feels he was seen by his GP for 'depression' treated with Diazepam.

Past medical history
Infantile convulsions. Nose bleeds before O-levels needed cauterisation with silver nitrate.

Mental state examination on admission
Appearance and behaviour
Stephen was appropriately attired and initially appeared to present well. However, there was some agitation evident and some bizarre behaviour, it was difficult to engage with him, he seemed preoccupied and changeable.

Speech – very low
Mood (O) Labile, perplexed, suspicious, fatuous
         (S) Not stated

Thought – possession – He appeared to have thought insertion. Little speech forthcoming, therefore? Thought blocking or withdrawal going on
Stream – Not continuous
Form – Evidence of disjointed incomplete form. Concrete thinking evident.
Content – Delusional, for example he thought he was a DNA isomer and explained how the whole room was in mirror images and it all emanated from the middle of the room, then looked very confused and at a later date thought members of staff were his parents and then again looked very confused and doubted if that was right.

Perception- Delusional perception evident? Visual hallucinations.

Cognitive functions – orientation – Not tested formally. However, he was not consistently orientated in time, place or person and his attention and concentration limited.

Provisional diagnosis – Psychotic episode (1)? Organic cause (2) Schizo affective

PART II

Please note – adverse reaction to Risperidone

----------------------- xxx -----------------------

25.6.97

Admitted this evening informally under care of Dr. M. Admitted direct from outpatients. 'Perplexed' as described by Dr M. Receives messages from the fourth dimension (time). NB. Is uninhibited. Within an hour of his wife departing TH was found by female nurse, naked and having just masturbated into his underpants. Did take 100mg CPZ after a little persuasion. It is my belief that he will need further persuasion to take more. I have asked him to keep himself decent when using his nurse call bell. I have explained to him that he is temporarily in a bed on the Mother and baby unit and will be moved as soon as is practicable.

'Is this (Rm 26) Earth'

'Can I be myself?'

'Is this the place to act out my fantasies?'

All of the above whilst standing in middle of the room stark naked.

Became more and more disturbed as the night progressed. Conversation more and more bizarre – very hard to ground.

'I am God'

'I am pleased when I see what I have done'

'You will not unravel the game, the sublime divine comedy.'

Repeated and spelt out, heaven, S—T and F—K over and over.

Occasional very loud and inappropriate behaviour/ laughter. Masturbating in front of me twice 'Only way I can get a vision.' Did stop when asked to. 100 mg CPZ at 0400 with little effect. Dr M has been notified re: above and has asked Dr B to see Steven as suggested increasing CPZ to 100 QDS. Also mentioned the possibility of the need to section.

26.6.97

Very confused and disturbed gentleman. Revealing bizarre and disjointed thoughts. No evidence of psychosis observed. Expressing desire to have sex with wife. 14th April and room 101 seem to be coming up quite a lot. Expresses regret for 'kill her sister in April.' I will die in the year 2000 at the Royal Albert Hall in room 101.

Urinalysis indicates negative. Bmstix 4 mmol/l % thirst and has drank about 4 litres of water. MMSE done on him and result as per chart Chlorpromazine 100 mg given with good effect. He has been in room all day, has a shower and in bed. Visited by wife this am and brother this pm. Became emotional and burst into floods of tears: re- 'Mum told me that a friend of hers died whilst they were on holiday' and he believes the friend mum was talking about was his father. He is however, for CXR and CT scan for further investigation.

Brother is concerned that something Steven had said indicated sexual contact with a gay friend. Brother queried need for HIV test. I explained that this could not be done without Steven's permission and he was not able to give informed consent.

Steven has had a much better night and the CPZ is having the desired effect. PAR obs disturbing him every time he is checked so suspended for most of the night. Sleeping at 0630.

27.6.97
Much more settled today, case plan discussed, Mood gradually became more elevated. Very surreal in conversation, lots of word association accompanied by episodes of thought block. Went out for a short escorted walk and displayed clear periods of apparent lucidity. On return to the unit proceeded to consume at least 7 litres of water. Continually rang his nurse call buzzer, though appeared to settle mid-morning.

28.6.97
At 0430 approximately he was brought yet another jug of fresh water and made sexually inappropriate suggestion then threatened to break her nose. Refused both oral Diazepam and Chlorpromazine. Dr Z contacted and requested to attend unit as Stephen then proceeded to break the plastic beakers in his room having ripped the nurse call box off the wall. Before Dr Z attended Stephen got dressed, packed some socks in a plastic bag and took his umbrella stating he was leaving the hospital. Very menacing and threatening. Kicked open side doors and left the

hospital. He proceeded in the direction of old Highlands where he broke into a staff member's car. Police called for assistance. Placed on section 52 Mental Health Act 1983 at 05.15. Wandered around the grounds for approximately one hour and then returned, ripping door handle off reception door. Reluctant to come back to unit. Restrained, hand cuffed and given Clopixol xxx 150 mgs intramuscular and Lorazepam 4 mgs intramuscular. Settled on return to room. Close observations maintained.

Stephen has slept soundly throughout the night. Seen by Dr Z who felt he was over-sedated, therefore no further medication to be administered. Fluids to be encouraged. For review.

29.6.97
Settled. Wife visited and they went out for a walk. He complains of sudden onset of headaches and sun reflects on his eyes and can't cope well without reflecting lens which his wife is going to get for him. Was in floods of tears regretting his behaviour on Friday and said he wants to get better but does not know what to do. Very frustrated but no evidence of aggression today.

Seen by Dr M this evening. Stephen appears calmer though continues to state his thoughts on being 'interfered with' – can have bad energies. Medication reviewed. Stephen has slept for the majority of the night.

30.6.97
Seen by Dr B to assess for a section 2 & Dr A appt @ 6.00 hrs.

Advised to limit his fluid intake which he has agreed to do. Remains perplexed and deluded. Thinks that the place is bugged and that the staff are actors who test him all the time.

Leaflet No 6 given. He has understood the meaning of his detainment and would like to appeal.

1.7.97

Quite calm. Went for Magnetic Resonance Imaging Scan at Pembury Hospital this morning. Found it very fascinating and would like to see the films from the scan when they are here. Wife came into visit and have spent most of the afternoon with him and he seems to be in a good mood.

Night

Polite and appropriate when engaged but did keep very much to himself. Awake at about 04.45 but settled back down with hot milky drink.

2.7.97

Quiet day. Visited by friend pm. Keeping very much to his room.

3.7.97

Quiet day. Walked to village. Viewed fitness room behaviour appropriate, no aggression. Wife visited this afternoon.

4.7.97

Quiet evening, received phone call from wife.

5.7.97

Had a settled day, less agitated and tense. Reviewed by Dr M who has written a section 17, at the discretion of staff, allowing him to go out. Has been visited at length by wife and has been out with her. Has been appropriate in mood and behaviour but still expressing some odd ideation.

Night
Request a walk for fresh air this evening and was allowed to sit in the garden for 15 minutes. Returned on time. Seemed totally appropriate tonight.

6.7.97
Almost ditto the above night entry. Pleasant, appropriate and settled. Short sit out in rose garden. Slept well.

7.7.97
Programme explained today. Steven felt he was well enough to join the programme. Appropriate but distant at times.

Walked to village with Steven this morning very pleasant and talkative.

Night
Seen by Dr M, discharged from Section 2. Very settled in mood. Appears to have slept well.

8.7.97
Support group – offered support to fellow patient. Said he felt less scrambled than admission. Requested a moment's silence at end of group.

Very upset by the window broken by other patient in his room.

9.7.97
Saw Dr M who finds Steven still somewhat perplexed but nonetheless much improved. May go home pm 10.7.97 for a couple of hours and overnight 12-13th if wife agrees.

10.7.97
All clear given. Went home by bus will return approx. 7.30pm depending on transport.

Returned about 7.30pm the visit had gone well.

11.7.97
Steven attended group- was appropriate, articulate.

Night
Sound asleep for most of the early evening. Pleasant and chatty while awake, watched TV and read until 10.30pm.

13.7.97
Returned from leave this evening stating he had had an enjoyable weekend and would like to go overnight leave during the week.

14.7.97
Totally appropriate. Commenced Risperidone 2mg curious about same but without suspicion. Has slept well.

15.7.97
Remains appropriate. Taking part in programme. No problem.
S/B Saw Dr M who asked me to go through the events of Steve's admission night. I did so but abridged the retelling somewhat. Stephen somewhat taken aback

but able to understand a lot of it. Appreciative of the session.

17.7.97
Quite appropriate on return from leave which he states went well. Complaining of itchy rash, reported to and seen by JB.

18.7.97
Very settled day, still complaining of rash, but very appropriate.

21.7.97
Returned from leave had been quite fragile at times.

22.7.97
Continues to complain of skin irritation. Seen by Dr M for discharge tomorrow – to have chlorpromazine and (xxx acti likewise PRN for TTOs).

23.7.97
Discharged 12.30 today.

Asylum

Difficult to tell the cared for from the carers, except
Where scars of razor cuts hash the lower arms.
I remember the day she came up to the window
Stared in at me from the garden, then battered
The panes with her wrists until the glass broke, drew
                                                    blood.

Carpeted corridors deaden sound, Georgian-wired
Fire doors, designed to resist heat
Partition means of escape - exits.
Precautions that seem to prevent
An outside threat from entering, not
Check the path of smoke, the spread of fire.

In this place, these lawns and gardens, time gathers,
Moments in sunshine, not having to think, a chance to
                                                    heal
For medication to stabilize. To be. And not to be afraid.

                            ***

White Lodge

I'd read about them sometime ago, their world famous,
alternative courses, healing, spiritual awareness. White
Lodge. I'd discovered that they do healing on Sunday
mornings - so I've come along. It's quiet, a peaceful
August Sunday. Ten o'clock. I enter the small chapel
first. I sit in silence, alone, staring into the beautiful, tiny
stained-glass windows tucked at the end of the tiny
white chapel.

When I come out there are people on the veranda
nearby, having coffee. I am the only one asking for

healing. An older man says he will help. He had been a spitfire pilot in the war. He stands behind the chair I'm sitting in. He rests his hands on my shoulders. His voice is even, steady, measured. He says I have a presence attached, someone who had been unable to leave this world. An elderly lady. I remember an old lady had died, a few years ago, in our new home, before we moved in. She had lived there most of her life. He says he will summon a welcoming party for her, in the spirit world...heaven. Then he simply offers her the opportunity to leave. I feel a weight being lifted. I am calm, peaceful. From that moment on things are clearer. A spitfire pilot. I understand. It makes sense. I will always be grateful to him. I owe him my life. I pay him nothing. He gives me his address, in case I should ever need to contact him again.

The laying of hands

The shadow stretches from behind the eyes
The length of the spine, peeling off the back
Of my head, a long-tailed reptile feeding
From the base of my brain. People stare past my eyes

They don't look at me, they only see the shadow
Lurking. I try to pretend everything is normal
Count the days of the week, the seconds spinning
I swing from tears to laughter, only gaining silence

Until with a fatherly hand he stands behind me
Holds my shoulders, conjures a reception party
And simply asks the spirit to leave.
There is the moment made fantastic as the energy

Subsides. I breathe again with friends, grateful

For this man's belief. He was a spitfire pilot
And has lost many friends, somehow he seems
To know what to do with demons.

***

Daily chores help to keep you grounded – earthed-
connected to the ground.

Mr Max
In my musings over the millennium, and during
recovery from my illness, I created a character called
Mad Max the Millennium Medicine Man who later
became...Mr Max the Mad Millennium Medicine Man.
He had a mop of shocking black hair and an evil
looking, green and silver painted papier mache mask
with a long hooked nose.

He became a character at a poetry slam in January
1999. He was born at The Common Dream an event
I'd organised to be all about Sustainable Development,
at the Forum in Tunbridge Wells near the autumn bank
holiday. Like Pumpkin Green. This had been the
forerunner for Groundswell. I'd hoped for hundreds but,
in the end, barely half-a dozen turned up.

The only reason we're here
Is that a few very big
And highly evolved monsters
Want us to be.

Watch how the shadow of a tree
Falls across an open field
Beneath the evening sun
Watch me balancing

Walking the tightrope
Between light and dark.

Skomer

We had two good holidays that summer while I was still away from work. The first with our son at a Field Studies centre in Pembrokeshire. Learning about the ecology of the area. One day was especially memorable for me. We took a boat trip out to the island of Skomer. Such a wild, bleak, barren place which had once been inhabited. Nature was there, raw in all her raging fury and beautiful in her tranquillity. My poem by the same name is also reminiscent of love. Of the presence of a former lover. And if you look more closely it is possibly even more introspective than that. A reflection of the changing internal moods and the love of the Muse.

Skomer

And the guttering red rock
Sliced like decks of cards
Slanted into the sea.

And she is there in the mist
In the sea breeze she
Is in the gathering dark
She rides the mounting forces
Which rise beneath the blackening waves
And she is in the quilted sky

She is there in the billowing
Sheeted veils of the afternoon
And in the rakish cry of the gulls

Screaming over the graves of shearwater
Skeletons, she is at the exits of hollowed burrows
Among bits of dead bird, dead rabbit, scattered
Beside the remains of Iron Age homesteads
And she is marking the way
In Celtic stone against the unforgiving grey.

***

La Rivolte
The second holiday was a writing week in the hillside
town of Grasse, renowned for its perfumes, near
Cannes and Nice. A week with Roger McGough, who I
knew from an Arvon Foundation writing course fifteen
years earlier. Unfortunately, still getting used to my
tablets, I was in bed early every night while the rest of
the group enjoyed the mild evenings, chatting in the
garden, playing pool in the bars.

31st August 1997
Coming down to breakfast on the Sunday morning,
there was a subdued silence among the three already
at the table. Princess Diana had died. The blanket fell
over the others as one by one they came down to eat.
A few days later, this simple poem was my response. It
is mixed with the emotion of one of the girls leaving
half way through the course without saying goodbye to
us.

Collision

Cut the red carpet
Shut up all the houses
Tear down the sides of the cradle

For she has died a young man's death.
I watched the Mercedes
Take her away
From under the shade
Of the pergola
No farewells
No chance to kiss goodbye
Only blood on the marble floor
And a faint sense of belonging.

A landmine ruptures in our heart
And all we have to offer are condolences.

1999

in which it is discovered that what goes around comes around…

Flow

Below. Above and beyond. Farther than your eye can see. Farther even than your deepest imagination. This magnificent sense of space which not only surrounds us but which lives within. Below the stars below the bubbling surfaces of the mind, the vibrations of the cortex, the tiny electrical, molecular impulses of the brain, to a place where you can chill, where your spirit even is at rest. A place of love… of consolation. A glorious space beyond the boundaries of death…

making connections matter.

4th January. I read an article in the Sun, entitled the 'Millennium itch'. It describes people's desires for new sexual experiences on the turning of Y2K. Sex in a lift. Sex in a plane. Sex with celebrities. Sex as the clock strikes midnight. Naughty, different, dangerous sex, at that precise moment.

A cluster of men in uniform with rakes, dragging them through the grass in the park, raking up twigs, moss.

19th February. We are experimenting with improvisation. I am on a drama course at the City Lit. We are learning about levels of tension that we can use in performance:

Level 1 – floppy, on the floor
Level 2 – stoned, barely standing
Level 3 – neutral, upright, alert

Level 4 – discovering, everything is new
Level 5 – directed, authoritative, determined (robotic)
Level 6 – fearful, paranoid, restless
Level 7 – extreme tension, fury, fear, shouting, explosive

Level 7 is the kind of tension you might feel if you are absolutely convinced that there is a live bomb in the room, one about to go off, and the exit is blocked. A situation I was later to believe.

First create being mud, lying flat on the floor, then start to bubble, energised, begin to rise, communicating with others through grunts and groans, becoming slightly more human, evolving...then starting again from the floor, becoming fire...fingers and toes beginning to crackle as paper and straw is lit, then wood...spluttering randomly into life...firing high, legs and arms flinging towards the ceiling, letting the voice be open, to roar...I discover through my fiery persona that I have become a fireman - I like to watch places burn.

While discussing fear with us, our teacher shares the following extract of a speech by Nelson Mandela:

Overcoming Fear

Our deepest fear is not that we are inadequate.
Our deepest fear is that we are powerful beyond measure.
It is our light, not our darkness that most frightens us.
We ask ourselves:
Who am I to be brilliant, gorgeous, talented and fabulous?
Actually, who are you not to be?

You are a child of the universe.
Playing small doesn't serve the world.
There is nothing enlightening about shrinking,
So that other people won't feel insecure around you.
We are born to make manifest the glory of the universe
Which is within us.
It is not just in some of us. It is in everyone.
And as we let our own light shine,
We unconsciously give permission
For other people to do the same.
And as we are liberated from our own fear,
Our presence automatically liberates others.

*By **Nelson Mandela.***

I later discover that it is attributed to Nelson Mandela's 1994, inaugural speech, informally on the lawns, and possibly cited from Marianne Williamson's interpretation of 'A Course in Miracles', in A Return to Love.

Friday 19th March 1999: *I appear on the Graham Norton show, reading out my 50 word story about Miles O'Keefe and Anne Robinson which he jokingly called shit. Even seven years later I meet someone who remembers seeing me then.*

Early that spring we went to Key West as a family. The long drive down the bleak Interstate 95 to the haven of brightly painted washboard houses in streets abundant with greenery. One night at midnight, walking back from the town having imagined I'd find some fun at Hooters, but it was closing, I felt as if I were being followed. I thought I might be murdered in these quiet streets, by knife or silenced gun. The next day, out snorkelling in thirty feet of water by the reef, I panicked when swimming back to the boat, we had drifted too far. I thought I was going to drown. It was all I could do to remain calm, to help my son back alive.

Not long after, in May, it happened again. Different circumstances and with little warning- quicker. The odds were against me. Apparently, a second time is quite common with some conditions.

We do not presume to come to this thy table, O merciful lord, trusting in our own righteousness, but in thy manifold and great mercies…

The Rutland Hotel.
I was on a visit to our organisation's Sheffield Association with one of my colleagues, a solicitor. We had travelled up by train from St Pancras the afternoon before. We had shared a bottle of Chianti in a wine bar that evening. I'm always wary of those bottles now. The ones shaped like a tall bulb, with raffia around the base.

***

His bedroom was narrow with a high ceiling. The kind of room made out of dividing up bigger rooms, where the plaster cornice disappears into the flat partition of a wall. The morning light seemed strange. He looked out of the window, noticed a Ross freezer lorry outside. We serve to please, said the strap-line. The design of the label seemed curious as if it were a front for some form of surveillance service. Other lorries were similar, like Coopers the bakers: Nothing is too much trouble, it said. Taking a shower, he read and re-read the message about the towels, and how the hotel wanted to take care of the environment.

There were more lorries passing the window as he ate his breakfast. There were a group of Americans waiting for their tour coach all sitting at one table. The leader glanced in his direction occasionally, exchanged some pleasantry. The man seemed to be keeping a secret from him. They began to move out. He felt they had been speaking in code.

He was to lecture on a course, an introduction to environmental issues. The technology of the laptop and the screen was superior to what he was used to. Everything was coded, on CDs. The course regularly referred to The Agency and instead of the Environment Agency he kept thinking of the CIA. The delegates were in short regimented rows facing him, as if they were at school. It seemed like a front for the army. He concluded that he was teaching the CIA to infiltrate companies as environmental advisers. Gradually he became aware that we might be in danger. There could be a bomb in the room. They could come under attack.

When he got on the train to head home he kept watching his back. He felt under threat. He walked most of the length of the train to find a safe seat. One where he had a good view of what was going on. A carriage that wasn't crowded. He chose a chair immediately in front of someone else. An older white-haired man. He thought at first that he could be garrotted from behind. So he turned sideways and spoke to him.

He was tense the whole journey. He felt trapped. He tried to talk casually to his neighbour behind him, as if he were in on the secret. He thought that the train itself might be a set up. He imagined the passing images of fields, telegraph poles, trees, roads, were just that, images projected on the sides of the train to pretend that they were moving. He thought it was a simulated journey. He laughed to himself because the projections were different on different sides of the carriage. Not realising that the views of either side are always different.

When he arrived at St Pancras and walked towards the huge clock face presiding over the platforms, he felt as if the army of passengers were protecting him as if he were on a gigantic film set, with hidden cameras recording everything.

His wife is away in Italy. He misses the Poetry Society evening. He grows scared of what or who is out to find him. He goes to bed early. The next day before his son goes to school, he sits him down in the hall and tells him that daddy has to go away but not to worry. Always remember mummy. I might be gone a while. I'm going to grandma and granddad's. To his son, then 10 years old.

He left, taking the car, flying up the A21 to Chelsfield. How he made the journey and survived without accident in such a state is more than surprising. At his parents, in their garden he played with the wedding ring on his finger. He'd lost so much weight that it would slide off his finger when he held his hand upside down. Previously he couldn't get it off at all. He kept turning his hand upside down, watching it slide off then putting it on the other hand and doing the same. It was only after recovering in hospital that he realised it had become fixed onto his other hand. As if it was only there for engagement.

The more I discover the less I know
The more I see the less I understand
The more I hear the less I know what to say
The more I touch the closer I become.

Still life

A silver, milk bottle top
Which I'm about to throw away
I look at it, partly crushed:
It's complex and contorted
Twisted surfaces, imagine
The mathematical equations
Which could describe its form.

Would any other top
With pressure equally applied, fold
Itself in exactly the same way?

       ***

The drug tipped me over the edge. 10mg Chlorpromazine which my father had obtained on prescription after speaking to my psychiatrist. The house is deep underwater, very deep. It is pressing in against the windows. The double glazing strengthened, quadrupled, to hold back the pressure of water. The windows are all sealed tight. My family are part of an experiment deep on the sea-bed. We have done something wrong. They are studying our behaviour. Studying how we have changed through childhood. How I have adapted. How I have coped with the changes. My parents regret some of the ways they brought us up, my brother and I. And I am here to learn.

I look through the centre of a crystal hanging in the front room window. It seems as if there is a tunnel of light running through it. Light which I can breathe. A tunnel of air, as if taking in a new breath. Later that night I imagine the house has filled with water, and I am wearing breathing apparatus. I have to get down to the front room to reach that air again. I move slowly. My Dad is walking with me, concerned that I am breathing loud and deep, that my breathing is forced through my teeth, as if I really am using the breathing apparatus which I imagine I have strapped to my back.

Torture. The reality so very frightening. It became real, not matchsticks beneath finger nails or electric currents, but surgical, without anaesthetic. It happened. I am lying on the bed, my arms, my feet shackled, tied down. The surgeon begins with a scalpel across my chest, searing pain. I scream, fearing what is to come. The operation begins, cutting deep, opening up the abdomen, methodically lifting, feeling, inspecting organs. I am still screaming. Wide awake.

The surgeon avoids the major blood vessels, runs the silver blade down the length of my legs and arms, revealing the folds of muscle. The skin drawn back. What are they expecting to find? The surgeon moves in on the heart, having prised apart the rib cage, split the sternum. Their faces are all looking down at me. I am hoarse from screaming, all my writhing, twisting, only tiny movements, looking up at their masks. The surgeon cups his hand around the beating heart. He lifts it out of its shelter, severing arteries. My final scream echoes the agony of all who have ever been tortured in the history of the world. Matching my last breath, it tails off, fades into a death rattle.

My father drove me to the hospital. (Shortly after he writes a poem on holiday with Mum in Ireland – The Burren, haunted by that final scream.)

The Burren [bhoireann – a stony place]
for Steve.

The road from Shannon to Ennis
Put us at ease, the inside lane
Marked for slow traffic and, strangers,
We took our time. In silences,
The mortar of marriage, we knew
Our thoughts were homing to you,
Sedated now, calm. Guilt easing
Under the miles to Mullaghmore
We were unprepared for the bare
Limestone, the alien uprising,
The scouring of land back to bone.

Only now, your scream in the night,
Explained - the agony of minds
Throughout time, in torment,
Searing through you - can the Burren
Be seen to have held your long howl.
That week it was right to walk out
From the cottage, breathe the release,
Putting aside the fear, the hurt
We felt for you, to step where glaciers
Had once scored rock, to study flowers.

That pavement, abundant with orchids,
Gentians, wood-sage, cat's foot, told

Of healing, of how the most barren
Of places recovers. Low cloud
Mimicked escarpments, softening
Harshness. Wells filled as we spoke
On the phone: you, yourself almost,
Echoes of cries in the dark
Diminishing, and we with a host
Of futures held in the Burren's past.

By **Ted Walter**

***

I had been more than reluctant to go to the hospital. I kept checking the car for bombs. Hardly dared to close the door in case I set something off. Dad had a friend follow in a car behind in case I caused trouble, grabbed the wheel, tried to run away. I sat in the passenger seat, my hands dancing as if I were doing tai chi movements, imagining that I was helping to drive, to steer the car, to change the gears. Believing that my dance was having an effect, could guide us to our destination. Ticehurst hospital. When I arrived I was still moving in tense Tai Chi style, not relaxed as you should be. I was in combat with evil spirits. As I moved swiftly in a spare room while waiting for another to be made up, I scared the male nurse looking after me. At the same time as my swift, silent movement the shower head fell off in the shower room with a loud bang.

Wednesday 26th May 1999
Ticehurst. Morning sunshine. Hesitant. Uneasy. Light sleep all night. Disorientated. I cannot imagine how people cope in war. Remembering all those executed for cowardice, for shell-shock, during the First World

War. Because this feels like a war. A war of nerves. Thrust and counter thrust. Balance, counter balance. Checking and re-checking the understanding of present. With and without drugs. A convoluted inner world.

Everyone grieves
the irretrievable landscape
of their childhood

MEDICAL NOTES
Date of Arrival 20th May 1999
Date of Departure 7th June 1999

Presenting complaints
Bizarre, threatening perceptions, 'signs of danger' everywhere – fear of death, fear of cancer, fear of bomb/fire/murders, premonitions, something trying to take over control (paranoid delusions, optic hallucinations).

Behaviour
Bizarre, paranoid, extremely tense and frightened, taking tai-chi like postures to keep away evil – still co-operative and able to engage in reflecting his state but hardly understanding it.

Speech
Low, insecure, frightened

Provisional diagnosis
Second psychotic episode
Paranoid schizophrenia

Final diagnosis

Schizo-manic episode

Most of the dreams were never realised, but they may be still...

28th June

He drives to meet his psychotherapist, his counsellor. She is to work with him over the next six years. On their first meeting he is in tears. With her he shares some of the most valuable time of his life. Connecting with what is real beneath the surface. Deep memories. Associations. Emotion. Beginning to understand. Helping to heal.

2000
in which the Millennium comes and goes…

Often, in the white interlaced knot of violent living being that swayed silently, there was no head to be seen, only the swift tight limbs, the solid white backs, the physical junction of two bodies clinched into oneness.
Women in Love, D.H. Lawrence

No celebrations in the Royal Albert Hall. A party at the Dome. Our street has a party, in and out of each others' houses. A smattering of fireworks. The New Year rises with the prospect of separation, of divorce.

October 2000
I trek the Inca trail, raising well over £2500 for the charity Whizz Kidz. My boss warned me to be careful about the altitude. Said it could affect me. I am still taking tablets. Olanzapine. On the trek I am on top of the world, so elated to be high in the Andes. On the last morning of the walk, we arrive at Inti Punku, the Sun Gate, overlooking the lost city. Our guide plays the Andean pipes and a condor comes into view circling high above us. It is a magical, spiritual moment. We stand in silence, listening, in awe.

Temple, Machu Picchu

She sits wearing her UCLA sweatshirt
Legs crossed, the forefinger and thumb
Of each hand touching, poised in meditation
Eyes focused at infinity
Beneath the stone wings of a condor.

She is perfectly aligned between mountains
The path of sun, moon, stars
Their tracks across the Earth
Known from some other time,
Before the white cloth of the Catholic Church
Fell, heavy with Inca blood.

2001

In which the new Millennium revisits the horror of the last...

And we have still not said enough. Not enough about consciousness...how life is, how it affects us, how we are what we are...what gives us soul, spirit, what it is that we strive for, those of us lucky enough to dream.

Tuesday 19th June 2001

At work, I attend the launch of working minds, the employer programme of mind out for mental health, a campaign to stop the stigma and discrimination surrounding mental health. I become what was rather grandly called an 'Ambassador' for the programme, agreeing to share my experience of mental ill health with a variety of audiences. Soon after I issue a press release on behalf of my employer in support of the campaign. I say:

'Employers cannot afford to ignore the problem of mental ill health which is set to affect an increasing number of employees. Bringing about a positive approach in the workplace and operating effective rehabilitation programmes is part of employment best practice and provides substantial business benefits.'

September 11th 2001

...we all share the pain of what happened this morning.

Birdsong

...as the stretcher- bearers lifted him, they turned his body and Stephen saw that the handsome face remained on one side, but on the other were the

ragged edges of skull from which the remains of his
brain were dripping onto his scorched uniform.[3]

Tall partners, almost identical, standing
Little more than a width apart, long legs, eleven.
The target of civilian, aerospace wings, glinting.

Where we once stood with millions
Looking out across the bay,
Swaying in the wind, over one thousand feet high.

The Towers melt like giant candles rapidly guttering,
Time-lapse sequences shifting
Beneath the horizon, clear blue, September sky.

How they implode floor by floor, one upon the other
Collapsing, as one falls the other follows swiftly after -
Flame tumbling with cloud, concrete, gypsum,
asbestos.

Bodies wick kerosene, are crushed, diced with glass,
with steel.
Beneath the rubble, through dust clouds, the tiny
violence of birdsong:
Mobile phones ringing, sequences of numbers seeking
loved ones, home.

***

November 2001
I have my appendix removed. Keyhole surgery. After
the pain has gone, it's amusing. Everyone has an

---

[3] *France 1916, from Birdsong, by Sebastian Faulks,*
published by Hutchison. Reprinted by permission of the
Random House Group Ltd..

appendix story to tell. I can chat about it happily without fear of stigma. I have not yet relaxed enough to chat about mental ill health. I recover with a picture of *Kylie* on my bedroom wall. Listen to my favourite tracks from her album. *Fever. Can't get you out of my head.* I have a poster of her in white, I cut out her shape in its entirety: high heels, breasts, raised microphone, neck, head thrown back. *Kylie* in song. I return to work fully after two weeks.

There are people in the park, running. A tall man jogging, flat footed. Leaves dance in front of car headlights, Horse-guards Parade. Already night at five o' clock. The rush hour queue of taxis leading up to Admiralty Arch, slowly edging through to Trafalgar Square...

2002
in which I revisit the holiday home...

January

Her face lit by the light of her mobile phone as she crosses the park as if she were looking into the face of the moon...

It happened again but quickly. He would burst into tears without warning. He sat on the edge of the bed before he was to go to hospital, trying to organise the business cards he had collected. Stacking them into piles. Who was important? Who wasn't? Who to follow up with on different ideas? He spread them out across the duvet. This might not seem unusual. But each decision, each choice was laboured, weighed, and each carried an overdose of emotion.

Something sinking in the pit of me, not communicating not breathing...

20.1.02
Steve was admitted at 16.30 hrs under the care of the consultant.
He slept almost the entire evening/night. Woke around midnight and showered. Watched some TV and went back to bed.

24.1.02
...this afternoon Stephen went out for a walk then attended tai chi, seems more talkative today.

28.1.02
Discharged to home address.

I am introduced to Lithium to help stabilise my mood. How strange to be swallowing this rare metal (in the form of lithium carbonate) to level the highs and the lows. Lithium, the lightest, silvery metal which, as I know from school, floats and burns on water and gives a crimson colour to a flame.

Moments when the particular experience - the random staccato of raindrops on his black umbrella at night, like radioactive disintegrations on a Geiger counter - awakens him to what is other than this earth...

I read how Julia Butterfly Hill camped at the top of a redwood tree, one hundred and eighty feet high, for two years to stop a massive logging programme. Somebody has to speak for the trees. (The Legacy of Luna. The story of a tree, a woman, and the struggle to save the redwoods, Harper SanFrancisco.)

2003

Bubbles float down the steel urinal in the Royal Oak, reflecting light in their meniscus, like tiny water boatmen, drifting...

Beech is regarded as the 'Mother of the Woods' for it is protective and nurturing, giving shade with its canopy and food that can be eaten in its raw state. As a large tree of the broadleaf forest it is also known as the 'beech queen' who stands beside the 'oak king'.
Jacqueline Memory Paterson, Tree Wisdom, Element.

How much would you pay for a back door?
I have seen hardwood doors for sale at only £50. But, I guess they were from unmanaged tropical rain forests. Summer 2003. They rang me. A cold call. I listened it seemed as if they were concerned. Are you worried about any aspect of the repair of your house? Your front door? No. Is your back door protected? No. I agreed. I felt unhappy about my back door. (Spot the subtle psychological reference!) There was a light dusting of mould. It was flimsy, dated. I agreed to speak to one of their sales reps. He rang me to say he'd be with me within the hour. Two hours later. He'd been held up along the way. He took details.

I opted for a loan. To supply and fit would be £1000. One thousand pounds! Somehow that seemed fair enough to me. I would have a pucker door. I'd feel safer. So they installed it - plastic coated with a double lock. Not long after, with inclement weather, water somehow found its way in. They kept calling on the off chance that I'd cave in again, sign up for some other crazy scheme. When I came to my senses I managed to pay off the outstanding loan and persuade them that I didn't want to hear from them again.

The girl working on her notebook smiles briefly as he squeezes past her on the train. The lace of her thong clearly visible above the waist of her jeans. He notices the small triangle of shiny material at the tail of her spine, the way it follows her curve...

I am interviewed for the Guardian, Jobs and Money and Business Breakfast TV. My story and how I was successfully brought back into work.

Stop the felling of the trees
August. I am playing *Evanescence* over and over again: *'Bring me to Life'*. I campaign to save trees in our local park. Magnificent, mature, tall cedars which are to be felled as part of a Lottery funded £2.3m improvement project. I start a petition. Over a hundred signatures in a few days. We are in the local newspaper. But the trees still come down. Gardening gone mad!

Rites of Passage.
Another men's' weekend. A course I had wanted to share for years. August 2003. The place set deep into the mountains of Wales, in the shadow of Snowdon. Cae Mabon. A traditional thatched roundhouse, full of the scent of wood smoke, covered with off-cuts of carpet and cushions all around the centre fireplace. A place for telling stories in a circle by the fire. Reliving stories. But I was taken to one side. They were not sure how the experience might affect me, since I'd just confessed to breakdowns in the first meeting.

Cae Mabon

In the shadow of Snowdon the encampment huddles
Among birch and oak, on a hillside facing Llanberis -
Home for eleven men surrendering to rites of passage.

I would have offered more had I known how deep
This could become, witnessing grief, hatred, anger,
                                                    love
Connecting through the symbols of grave, effigy,
                                                    sword.

But I confessed to my daily splitting of foil, for tablets to
                                                    balance
The highs and the lows, bringing me to a level
Tender place, and they offered to protect me from the
                                        ravages of spirit.

So very real the moment he stamped on her effigy,
                                                    destroyed
Her among the ashes of the hearth, or he cried over
Turned earth, or he raised the sword in anguish,
                                        repentance.

In the roundhouse he marked the next steps of his life
                                                    journey
With the heart of an oak, a lion, we saluted
His marriage to come, his future family, completely in
                                                    love.

In our unity time dissolves, we find grace as men
                                                    bound
To each other, embracing our experience of the other
                                                    side
Which is within ourselves - learning to share the
                                        eternal.

For one of the group we recreated a burial. I helped to dig the grave. For his father. For him to reconnect with his grief- to learn. I was no mere spectator after all. None of us were. We became witnesses. We shared in the man's pain and supported him though his rite of passage. He cried. But came through healed.

For me, they gave me time just to sit up in the hillside to write. For my ritual they listened intently, honestly, to my poems. I could not have wished for a better audience. I felt stronger. Relieved. Overjoyed.

25th October
I drop into your life like an acorn… ask you out.

6th November
Our first date together…

2004
in which I am discharged for the last time…
maybe…

This is coach number 1 of 11, the automated voice says confidently, when the guard has just told us there are only 7 coaches, to which all who are standing will testify.

March
Making love in the Old Ship Hotel, Brighton. A new, deeper love. Mingle mangle.

July
We return from a wedding in Burgandy. My lover discovers her colleague physiotherapist has bowel cancer, her brother in law dies, her daughter is in trouble with the local shopping centre, and I end up in hospital.

26.7.04
To Dr A from Dr M

Steve was discharged from TH on Friday 23.7.04. He was admitted on 19.7.04. He had started to experience ideas of suspiciousness and a delusional mood feeling that there was something going on around him. He had also become emotionally labile with bouts of crying. At times his thoughts had also been racing.

I was concerned that he had relapsed into a Mixed Affective Episode. We agreed for a brief admission and he has been stabilised on Olanzapine 10mg at night and Lithium Carbonate 1200mg at night and Lorazepam 1mg at night. His mood had appeared to have stabilised significantly and he was adherent with recommended medication. There were slight concerns that he was still suspicious before he left, but he left with his partner... and she was aware of the risks and agreed to contact us if there was a problem.

He was given one week's supply of medication to take away. In addition to the psychotropic medication, he also takes Ezetrol (Ezetimibe) 10mg at night.

I will see him at the Nuffield in just over a week's time and I have told him to contact me in the meantime should he get into difficulty.

Dr. M.

The steamy La Senza poster at Charing Cross station. Perfectly formed buttocks, dressed only in a lace thong. See how his mind races even among the grey river of commuters at nine in the morning. To slip inside cunt, beautiful cunt, slick, soft, heavenly cunt. Fuck, fuck, fuck...

Travelling home, deftly he undoes the multi-coloured foil wrapper of a Cadbury's Crème Egg without making a tear, gently bites off the cap and pushes his tongue deep inside, licking it out, thick, rich, creamy...

2005
in which I am not a patient...

Images of the closing scenes in snow of Farenheit 451, the temperature at which books burn, by Ray Bradbury. People living in the woods to escape the society in which no books are allowed, and any discovered are burned. They become their favourite novels, reciting for younger ones to learn.

Monday 25th July
I'm invited to a reception at Downing Street. I get to shake hands with Tony among two hundred other people who've done something for their community. My contribution, a few presentations - baring my soul.

August
I revisit Ticehurst out of curiosity. On the picnic table in the rose garden a dehydrated daisy chain. I flick through the blue card files in the office - like surveyors' reports on houses, assessing their structural integrity - psychological reports on me, assessing integrity of mind.

Simply the peace. To be protected. To let the mind settle. To come off the boil, the fear, released by chlorpromazine, the valve on a pressure cooker. In the garden the soft lawn. Privacy behind the hedges, trellises, two tall round fir trees in the centre, a border of rhododendrons, roses.

This place, where they cared and observed, observed and cared for me but seemed to know little about the inner world, the psychic turmoil. Sitting within the shade of the tall cypress tree. The greenfinch persisting with its plain monotonous repeated buzz.

Chaffinch. Song thrush. Blackbird. Wren. Listen to them sing.

The visitor

Lichen on the picnic table
A dehydrated daisy chain
Shrivelled like fine fragments of coral

The same stillness, the same birdsong,
The white house bathed in sunshine, masking
Tormented worlds, the aggregation
Of years of fear, misunderstanding, confession.

The parts we never saw, the offices,
Residential accommodation, kitchens,
Upstairs where they treated victims of head injuries.

Now they will no longer pay for me to be here – it's time to leave.

***

An oak leaf falling, kisses him on the cheek, stays with him as he walks into the breeze…

I also revisit Braeside. Pembury Hospital Mental Health Services. The consulting rooms are in shabby huts. White plastic weatherboarding, asbestos roof tiles heaped with tufty green lumps of moss. First the psychiatrist takes a history. Then recommends that I return in three months.

Perhaps we sometimes see glimpses of what is truly real, which is far greater than our day-to-day experience might have us believe. But sometimes even the simplest, plainest routine experiences, such as doing the washing-up, enable us to connect with something of the eternal.

Washing up, drying up and putting away

Dad places a steaming wet plate
Into the drying rack
For me to wipe up and put away.

He continues talking galaxies:
Did you know that light from the farthest stars
Has travelled so far
It left them before the earth was born?

Thirteen billion years.
That we should be here at all -
Creatures of time and space –
Is miracle enough. And yet
We share a foothold with some other dimension.

I dry the dinner plate, slide it in on top of others
Then wait beside the sink for cups and saucers.

***

2006

in which I am found to be euthymic…

The sun rises. In that short phrase, in a single fact, is enough information to keep biology, physics and philosophy busy for all the rest of time.
Lyall Watson, Lifetide, © Lyall Watson 1979, Hodder Headline.

For the next visit my notes had been typed up: my very own neat, new folder. Three monthly checks. To see me. To ask me how I am. To check on my demeanour. The same interval as the lithium blood tests should be. Checking for electrolytes, blood count, kidney and liver function. Thyroid function, every six months. You need to be stable on this medication for sometime she says.

24th February 2006

Dear Dr A,

Re: Stephen Walter d.o.b 1960
Tunbridge Wells

I saw Mr Walter in the outpatients' clinic at Braeside on 22 February 2006.

He stated he was doing well and he did not report any problems or side effects from the medication except weight gain. He stated he was coping well with everything and was enjoying his work. He said that he had normal duty hours at work and was under no special treatment.

He was casually dressed, maintained good eye contact and rapport was established. His mood was subjectively and objectively euthymic. His speech was spontaneous and coherent with normal rate, volume and flow. There was no evidence of any thought disorder or perceptual abnormality. His cognition was intact and he had good insight into his mental state.

He will continue on lithium 1200 mgs nocte and Olanzapine 7.5 mgs nocte. I will review him in 3 month's time. I would be grateful if you could do his serum lithium levels and renal function tests every 3 months and thyroid function test and full blood count every 6 months.

Yours sincerely,

Dr J.

Walking… more aware of the weight of his balls, his cock folded tight in the pouch of his pants.

The Royal Oak

Dark, lacquered panelled walls, a walnut piano,
The landlord pumping bitter - real ale. Black Sheep.
I drank here with my brother before his wedding.

For you, Chilean Merlot - the landlord's favourite.
I choose Guinness, Extra Cold. Outside, the sign
                                                    hanging
From a dead branch swings and squeaks. Long past
                                                    time
To plant an acorn, sapling. Dethroned, a lone stump

Of a tree, its bark splitting, peeling, fungus eating in.
Drinking… music from the sixties repeating.
Riding the tension of the Ashes - the landlord's
favourite.

Our usual seats: you ask me if I know what it's like
To burst into tears when someone shows you
kindness.
So much you wish you could have changed.
I love you as the sun blazes, blasts colour through the
windows.

***

*You have to be aware that there will always be a
vulnerability there…*

*There never was a before
Not after this
There never could be…*

*Sunlight filters through the slats of partly open, wooden
shutters casting shadows on the wall's fractured ochre
plaster…*

*The peace of God, which passeth all understanding,
keep your hearts and minds in the knowledge and love
of God, and of his Son Jesus Christ our Lord: and the
blessing of God Almighty, the Father, the Son and the
Holy Ghost, be amongst you and remain with you
always. Amen.*

And to close, quite a different form of veneration…

In the Navy

They've erected a scaffold all the way up
Lord Nelson's column, a sheath of boards, poles
And netting over one hundred and fifty feet high.

He's stood there for more years than his height
Measured in feet. What's going on behind this thin,
Blue veil at the centre of London?

They are cleaning every inch meticulously
A little favour for the old sailor -
Fellatio on a colossal scale!

***

...stand behind the yellow line!

EPILOGUE

The experience I describe of being offered up onto the operating table without anaesthetic, is a little like sharing these secrets.

My only hope is that being open about my experience of madness might encourage others to be more open too, so that we may all discuss mental health freely and without stigma.

It would be good if awareness of mental health became an accepted part of the everyday, like: 'How are you?'

Steve

Appendices

M^{c}M

Extract from a presentation on monitoring disability, to the Employers' Forum on Disability conference, The Churchill Room, HM Treasury, 17th November 2005.

So let me introduce myself again, properly: Steve Walter, BSc DipEH MBA CMIOSH RSP CEnv H,S&E Adviser, Born 1960, National Insurance Number WZ 85 43 77 Y, Diagnosis: bipolar affective disorder, currently 1200 mg Lithium and 7.5 mg Olanzapine, daily at night. So is this me? Is this the sum total of who I am? Simply another statistic labelled disabled? I wasn't disabled before 1997 but apparently I am now.

Of course, I could have been replaced here today a thousand times over. There are so many who have suffered mental health problems, but fewer perhaps who have, so far, been successfully rehabilitated back into work.

Mine is one of many 'stress-related illnesses.' While pressure can help to stimulate inspiration and ideas, excessive pressure can cause stress, and when sustained, stress destroys creativity and harms mental health.

In many ways I am still trying to make sense of what I have experienced. Some moments were very positive, others very frightening which I wouldn't wish on anyone.

My diagnoses have been mixed. I now know that there are few black and white cases of mental ill-health. I certainly didn't want to hear schizo-affective disorder. However, last year I asked an audience, who had been diagnosed with bipolar affective disorder such as my self, how many had also been diagnosed at some stage with schizophrenic symptoms like me and at least a third held up their hands. This was very reassuring – to know I am not the only one. Of course it is a truism to say that it is not the diagnosis that counts it is the person. However, this can be forgotten in the rush to put a monitoring system in place.

Stigma and mental health
Strangely perhaps, although I have published and given presentations discussing some of the main circumstances surrounding my breakdowns, and have discussed them with close friends, I have not shared them widely at work, hardly at all. I still sense a kind of taboo, a discomfort or unpleasantness surrounding mental ill-health, and who I might talk to, and this discomfort is not least on my part.

Even the phrase 'mental health' has associations for some with Victorian Asylums for the insane, although this is changing.

'How do I cope with the label 'disabled'? By its very definition this label is the opposite of enabling. How do I handle the stigma? What do fellow employees think of as disabled? If I am asked 'Do you consider yourself to be disabled?' My first reaction is NO! Because I do not feel disabled most of the time. It comes back to the spectrum of mental health on which we all shift our positions day to day. No - I might say – I'm not disabled how dare you expect me to say that I am?!

My gut response is that I do not want to be labelled to be pigeon holed, numbered, categorised, catalogued, dehumanised and possibly discriminated against. I f****ing hate it. It makes me so angry. People's assumptions and presumptions about me, my personality, my abilities. It is annoying enough being asked questions by a car hire company when they see that my driving licence, although valid, is up for review in two years and they ask why. And I have to say because of the drugs I'm taking or again use that horrible word 'medication'.

But while I imagine that I'm perfectly capable I realise I'm not, not without drugs -too much stress and I flip into another world. I have had to come to terms with the fact that I have an occasionally repeating illness for which I need to take medication. If I didn't have the drugs then I would, probably more readily, recognise myself as disabled because the symptoms would be evident.

But when I had my appendix removed, a few years ago, it was a completely different story. I chatted to everyone about it. Everyone had an appendix tale to tell - and were more than happy to! There was no stigma attached.

Perhaps part of the reason for my personal sense of stigma surrounding mental ill health is that I often view it as a kind of failure, a weakness, much more so than a simple injury would be.

May I leave you with this thought which hints at another aspect of the nature of experience?

When we stand against the backdrop of the universe and turn to face eternity, we may glimpse what spirit is.

I have summarized my experiences and how we managed my return to work in more detail in the personal case studies section of the HSE's stress website: *http://www.hse.gov.uk/stress/personal.htm*

I hope I have given some insight into the possible implications of monitoring. You may be interested in my personal website which has the links to more details of my experiences.

www.makingconnectionsmatter.org

Reflecting on Chris Moon
Unlike someone who has suffered and overcome major disability like Chris Moon, who was blown up by a landmine and lost his right arm and leg, I have not suffered in the face of bravery. I simply bear the wounds and battle scars of everyday life.

www.chrismoon.co.uk

MAKING CONNECTIONS MATTER

This appendix describes what making connections matter is all about. It occupied my mind for much of the time from 1995 to 1997 and ever since. The following pages include extracts from the website www.makingconnectionsmatter.org

Welcome to *making connections matter*, inspired by the human condition on planet earth. *Making connections matter*, draws on experience. It is a personal brand with several meanings:

- the infinite becoming finite, spirit becoming real
- M^{c}M* is a huge number, extra-universal
- creative thought, poetry, bringing ideas to life
- mind making sense of the reality we think we know
- bridging the millennium, 1900 (MCM) through the present, to 2100
- connections spanning centuries, grandparents, parents, child.

It is also about linking people concerned for the environmental and humanitarian impact of their purchasing decisions.

*M^{c}M is a representation of the logo. As Roman numerals, if read simply as MCM, it stands for the year 1900. But if read as in the logo as a mathematical expression (with the lower case italicised 'c' representing 100, raised as a power, and the M representing 1000 and also multiplying), it becomes a very large number (1000 multiplied by 1000 one hundred times, multiplied by another 1000 - it works out to ten to the power of 303 - that's 1 with three hundred and three zeros after it!!!). In this appendix you'll discover that M^cM is a bigger number than you may at first think.

As well as being a mega number, M^cM is also the abbreviation for 'making connections matter' which is about inspiration, creativity, bringing ideas, arising in thoughts - connections in the brain - to life. Making Connections Matter derives from the connections which exist between all living things since the origins of time and space.

Connections spanning centuries, grandparents, parents, child
The roots of M^cM for me go back to my grandparents, born around 1900 (MCM). Most of us remember our grandparents, some our great or even great, great grandparents. There are profound connections through families, from grandparents, to parents, then to yourself as a child, through to your children and your children's children.

If all is well in life, you may know everyone of these generations within your own family. Current, younger generations have bridged the millennium (MM) and our grandchildren, especially if they are yet to be born, may survive through to the turning of the next century 2100 (MMC).

Often it seems that this link through generations continues even after death. *Making connections matter* is also about this connection between the spirit world and the material world, through those who are known, especially family, our own flesh and blood, connecting with us in spirit. And our friends, close friends, linking through spirit to greater love.

Making connections matter - **spirit becoming real.**
While M^{c}M was growing with me in 1997 I took inspiration from my dead grandparents (especially my maternal grandmother) as if I were tapping energy from a source outside of myself, as if it were spirit bringing a deeper understanding of life.

For me *making connections matter* is about keeping a clear perspective on reality while being inspired through connecting with the eternal, profound moment of existence. It is about spirit in a material world.

Often at the point of breakdown, although frightening at times, it is as if I am more open to the source of my creativity, my Muse. Much of what I have written about, in terms of creativity and connections, came alive, was energized during this profound psychological disturbance, setting the world in an even deeper spiritual context.

Creativity. To be inspired, to be moved by art, beauty, winning performance, dance, music, painting, sculpture, writing, even articulating dissent, the human voice, the human body, ecstasy, heights we aspire to...

Making connections matter is primarily about creativity - spirit becoming real, bringing ideas (thoughts which seem to come out of thin air) to life. Inspiration is, in a sense, matter (the real, conscious mind) connecting with spirit (the Muse, the source of inspiration) and then spirit becoming matter, becoming real through the new idea. Imaginative spirit, bringing ideas to life.

As I have shown, I work to bring ideas to life through poetry. I also value the power of performance, of theatre, of poetry being brought alive without the written page.

The Common Dream

Most of us desire a comfortable life, one of convenience, all the food we need or want easily accessible in nearby shops, everything on tap - heat, water, light.

However, everything we choose to do, and in particular what we buy, is connected to some environmental and humanitarian impact. While it may be of immediate benefit at the point of consumption (providing food, drink, helping the economy etc.) there are usually associated negative impacts, such as waste.

Whether it's wood taken from tropical rainforests, that has been felled without any attempt to manage and minimize the ecological damage, or products in excessive packaging, or meat from animals that have been intensively reared with no access to the open air, perhaps fed residue from carcasses of the same species (the underlying cause of BSE) - animals treated like vegetables, with no chance to experience a real life.

We need to be aware of where our food and other products have come from. To know their roots, how they arrived in the shops, or came to be delivered to our door – *making connections matter*. We cannot continue to isolate ourselves from the reality of what we choose to do, what we choose to buy.

We need to be aware of the very real connections between our choices and the related impacts on the ecology of the planet. To recognize and respect the connections between ourselves and every other living being, connecting with the natural rhythms of the earth, and ultimately, our place in the universe.

We could become stewards rather than consumers, to help sustain rather than destroy, the diversity, beauty and abundance of life on earth.

For a selection of related websites which can give more information on the ethical implications of purchasing visit www.makingconnectionsmatter.org.

The infinite becoming finite

M^{c}M represents the infinite as a huge number becoming finite, expressed as three simple letters - as spirit becomes flesh through conception and birth so ideas are brought to life.

M^{c}M is a huge number, consider for example:
- M^{c}M is a mega number
- How many times does a human heart beat in a lifetime?
- How many people on the planet?
- How many red blood cells in the body?
- How many neural connections in the brain?
- How many seconds in the life of the earth?
- How many stars in the universe?
- How many atoms in a teaspoon of carbon?
- How many atoms in the universe?
- What is a googol?
- What is a googolplex?

M^{c}M is a mega-number

M^{c}M is, as these examples show, extra-universal. In one sense it is a measure of time: A millennium to the power of a century, multiplied by a millennium (or

1000^{100} 1000 or 10^{303} (ten to the power of 303) years). This is many, many times greater than the age of the universe (which is estimated to be only 15 billion or 1.5×10^{10} years old).Remember 1000 is 10x10x10 or 10^3 .

Here are some other natural numbers which show the scale of M^{c}M.

How many times does a human heart beat in a lifetime?

The 'least shrew' from America weighs between 2-2.5 grams. A least shrew's heart beats about 400 times per minute and can even go as high as 1,000 beats per minute while an elephant's heart rate is just about 25 beats per minute with a heart that can weigh over 28 pounds. A female blue whale has been recorded with a heart that weighed 1540lbs (698.5kg) - that's nearly three-quarters of a ton!

The human heart beats an average of 70 times per minute. In a lifetime of 80 years that means the heart beating about 42,048,000 or 4.2×10^7 times.

How many people on the planet?

There are about 6.4billion (6.4×10^9) people on the earth.

How many red blood cells in the body?

There are 25 billion (or 2.5×10^{10}) red blood cells (these cells carry oxygen) in the average human body.

How many neural connections in the brain?

The human brain has about 100 billion neurons. Estimates of the number of synapses (the numerous connections between neurons) have been made in the range from 10^{13} to 10^{15}.

How many seconds in the life of the earth?
The Earth has been around for about 4.5 billion years, about 1.4×10^{17} seconds.

How many stars in the universe?
There are far too many stars for scientists to count, but by estimating, scientists believe that number of stars exceeds 1,000,000,000,000,000,000,000 (10^{21}). There are more stars in the universe than there are drops of water in the oceans of the world or grains of sand on all the beaches of the earth.

How many atoms in a teaspoon of carbon?
This is something known as Avogadro's number - 6×10^{23}. It is the number of atoms in an equivalent weight to the atomic weight in grams (also known, rather curiously, as a mole). For example the atomic weight of carbon is 12.
There are approximately 6×10^{23} atoms in 12g of carbon. More than the number of stars in the universe.

How many atoms in the universe?
How many atoms in a star? Let's say the Sun is a typical star and it's made up totally of hydrogen. The mass of the Sun is estimated to be around 2,000,000,000,000,000,000,000,000,000,000kg (2×10^{30}). The mass of a hydrogen atom is 0.00000000000000000000000000017kg (1.7×10^{-27}). Divide one by the other and the number of atoms in the Sun is about:
1,200,000,000,000,000,000,000,000,000,000,000, 000,000,000,000,000,000,000 (1.2×10^{57}).

Now multiply that by the number of stars in the universe and you have: 1 with 77 or 79 zeros after it (depending how you do the calculation).

Another way of doing the sum is to take the mass of the observable universe as 1 with 52 zeros after it kilograms. It's thought that's about 90% of the total mass of the universe which is then estimated to be 10 with 52 zeros after it kg. Divide that by the mass of a hydrogen atom (the vast majority of the universe is hydrogen) and the number of atoms is 6 with 79 zeros after it.)

There are approximately 6×10^{79} atoms in the universe. (Much less than M^cM).

What is a googol?
The name 'googol' was invented by a child (Dr Kasner's nine-year-old nephew) who was asked to think up a name for a very big number, namely, 1 with a hundred zeros after it. A huge number but by no means infinite. At the same time that he suggested 'googol' he gave a name for a still larger number: 'Googolplex'.

A googol is 1 with 100 zeros after it or 1×10^{100}.

M^cM (1000^{100} 1000) is even bigger than a googol. M^cM is big enough to embrace all of the above numbers many times over, except for the googolplex.

What is a googolplex?
A googolplex is much larger than a googol, but is still finite. Apparently, it was first suggested that a googolplex should be 1, followed by writing zeros until you got tired. But different people get tired at different times! The googolplex then, is a specific finite number,

with so many zeros after the 1 that the number of zeros is a googol.

A googolplex is much bigger than a googol, much bigger even than a googol times a googol. A googol times a googol would be 1 with 200 zeros, whereas a googolplex is 1 with a googol of zeros!

You will get some idea of the size of this very large but finite number from the fact that there would not be enough room to write it, if you went to the farthest star, touring all the nebulae and putting down zeros every inch of the way.

A googolplex is $10^{100^{(\times 100)}}$). (Ten to the power of a hundred to the power of a hundred.)

A googolplex is many times bigger than $M^\circ M$

With thanks to the site on Google which lists the googol.

What can we do to make a difference?
What can we do to make a difference? ...How do our everyday choices really affect the planet? ...Do we believe that they can? This 'story' is an extract from a pilot radio programme considering our impact on the planet.

When I was younger, my brother and I used to help an elderly, blind friend of the family with the gardening, decorating and odd jobs. She was a delightful woman, Marie. She was quick-witted, intelligent and generous. Over some summer holidays, as a student, I used to read to her. She was particularly keen on books by Lyall Watson, and I remember clearly reading all of his fabulous Supernature, and Lifetide over consecutive summers, by the caravan in her garden in sunshine. If you know the books, I think you'll agree that Lyall has the ability to bring apparently disparate things together, to allow us to marvel at nature in all of her mysterious connections. Marie was fascinated by his descriptions of the unusual, the miraculous in nature, and would despair at Man's exploitation of the planet.

If you're like me you'll care passionately about our home, planet earth. It grieves me that the everyday things I do damage the environment: consuming energy, contributing to waste, from the moment I flush the loo, switch on the kettle, travel to work, buy my weekly shopping, my ecological footprint is stamped all over the earth. And there are millions like me, like you. Together we would need several more Earths for us all to sustain our current standard of living. For the whole world's population this could mean over four more Earths (see www.myfootprint.htm). We cannot continue consuming resources, and wasting so much as we do now. It is not sustainable.

Some time ago I wrote to my local supermarket - well, all my local supermarkets in fact -about an apparently silly thing...I'd noticed that more and more of the bottles of wine I bought, and I was buying a lot of them (!) had plastic corks. Now sometimes little things can seem particularly annoying. Why? Why plastic corks, what's wrong with natural cork? Perhaps it's better that they're not cutting down the cork trees, I thought, naively. Then I noticed a newspaper article about a campaign by the RSPB (the Royal Society for the Protection of Birds).

Apparently they had been campaigning for a couple of years. Their website (www.rspb.org) is full of useful information including a report they'd commissioned - 'the Cork report.' I discovered that the increased use of plastic could have serious damaging effects on Europe's natural cork forests in Spain and Portugal.

Many species of birds and animals rely on healthy cork forest for food and shelter and the forests also contribute to the local economies. If the natural cork industry declines, species such as the booted eagle, black kite and turtle dove could disappear from large areas of Spain and Portugal, along with many other already threatened animals and plants.

Natural cork is a truly sustainable product (since it's taken from the bark and the trees keep on growing) and its one which benefits people and wildlife. The Iberian cork forests have taken thousands of years to develop but it will take only a few years for them to disappear.

And, unwittingly, I am responsible for increasing the market for plastics and threatening these forests because I am buying the wine! I wrote to the supermarkets not only to challenge the policy of using plastic corks but also to ask for the choice. How can I tell what types of cork are used unless the bottles are labeled? Since then, M&S at least have taken to labeling their wines in this way, identifying where synthetic corks are used.

As the North American Indian, Chief Sealth, or Seattle as he is now known, is reported to have said in 1854:
The earth does not belong to man; man belongs to the earth. This we know. All things are connected like the blood which unites one family. All things are connected.

Whatever befalls the earth befalls the sons of the earth. Man does not weave the web of life, he is merely a strand in it. Whatever he does to the web, he does to himself.

These connections matter. The connections between what we choose to do and the future of life on the planet matter – making connections matter. In future pages we'll consider the links between our lives and the planet. We'll talk about our choices and their impacts on others and on the planet, on product life cycles, and much more. We'll hear how some peoples' choices really have made a difference and I'll take you back to that sunny garden reading the wonders of Supernature. Do join me again.

Messages...

We know that the emptiness of space is a fullness far beyond our comprehension; that the nature of black holes is to produce, that the apparent 'no-thing-ness' is poised to create. This is where all life originates, bubbling into being. Spirit requiring an embodiment to speak its name. Spirit, at the heart of darkness, does not know darkness but, once embodied it strives for light, fearing an extinction that it need not fear, for everything returns to the positive darkness wherein it can 'see'.

Only our embodied eyes have learned to fear the dark. In creative spirit darkness and light are all one. On our paths we meet and know this oneness, but our social order, our transient rules, restrict the voices that wish to sing our joy at the discovery of shared beginnings. Fear not the dark, the emptiness, for from it births the truly creative spirit and love knows this, love would have all beings know it.

Ted Walter.

***

Of nebulae…

Hearts and Minds
mystifying
perplexing at times
trying to find words for words
which was just a feeling
a nebulous cloud to walk through
now and again the sun shone
and its rays filtered inside
on to the green chakra
like a long smile
with joy

Hazel Walter

***

Quoting from **Mary Baker Eddy…**

All is infinite mind in its infinite manifestations

Marie Barrett *(deceased).*